Strategies
Health Care Worker Fatigue

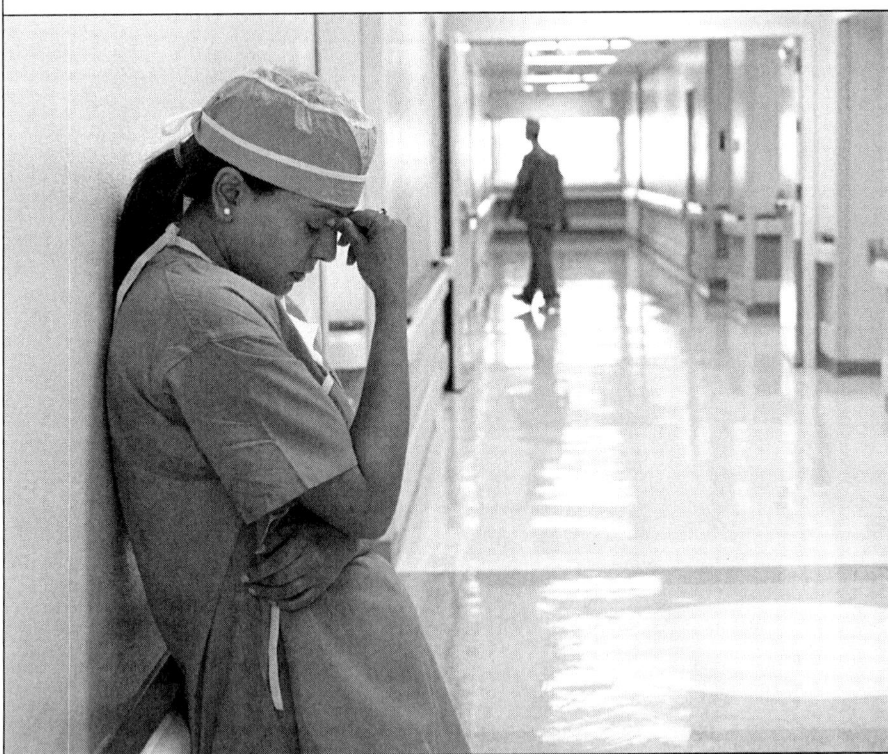

The Joint Commission

Senior Editor: Audrie Bretl
Project Manager: Bridget Lillie
Manager, Publications: Paul Reis
Associate Director, Production: Johanna Harris
Associate Director, Editorial Development: Diane Bell
Executive Director: Catherine Chopp Hinckley
Vice President, Learning: Charles Macfarlane, F.A.C.H.E.
Joint Commission/JCR Reviewers: Patricia Adamski, Deborah Nadzam, Kelly Podgorny, Paul Reis

Joint Commission Resources Mission
The mission of Joint Commission Resources is to continuously improve the safety and quality of care in the United States and in the international community through the provision of education and consultation services and international accreditation.

Joint Commission Resources educational programs and publications support, but are separate from, the accreditation activities of The Joint Commission. Attendees at Joint Commission Resources educational programs and purchasers of Joint Commission Resources publications receive no special consideration or treatment in, or confidential information about, the accreditation process.

Printed in the U.S.A. 5 4 3 2 1

Requests for permission to make copies of any part of this work should be mailed to
Permissions Editor
Department of Publications
Joint Commission Resources
One Renaissance Boulevard
Oakbrook Terrace, Illinois 60181
permissions@jcrinc.com

ISBN: 978-1-59940-229-1
Library of Congress Control Number: 2008928655

For more information about Joint Commission Resources, please visit http://www.jcrinc.com.

Contents

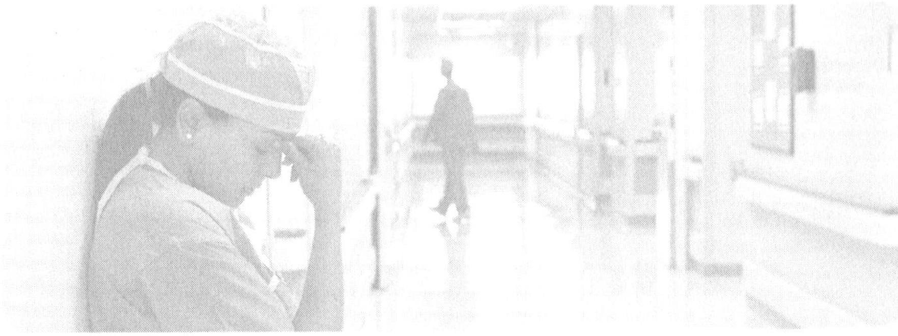

Introduction

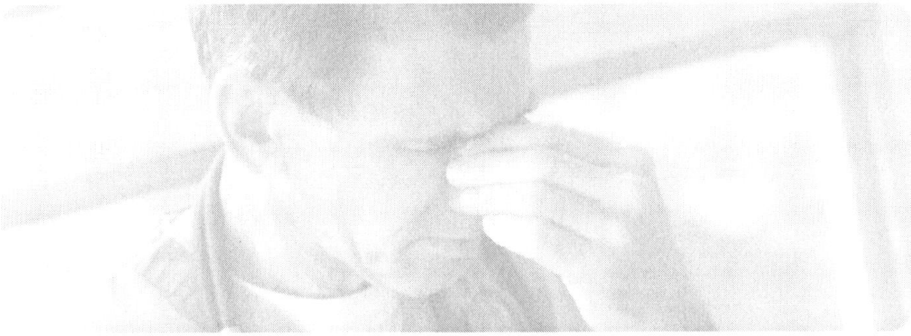

A 43-year-old patient enters a hospital expecting safe, high-quality care. What she does not know is that her physician has not slept in 24 hours; the nurse's shift ended 4 hours ago, but she was asked to work overtime because of a staffing problem; and the pharmacist preparing the patient's medications hasn't been sleeping well at night due to stress at work. Will the care this patient receives be the best it could possibly be? Probably not. Will someone make a mistake? Can an error occur? Possibly.

Worker fatigue and burnout in health care organizations are serious problems that can affect both patient and staff safety. Due to the continuous nature of health care delivery, many organizations require their workers to engage in long hours, overtime, and shift work that can occur during non-daytime hours. Consequently, many health care workers often report to work tired and/or experience extreme fatigue while on the job. Long periods of high stress, lack of sleep, and continual interaction with people who are sick—many of whom may not recover—can lead to worker burnout. The consequences of fatigue and burnout among health care workers can be severe. An individual worker can experience significant health effects, such as depression, hypertension, and an increased risk for cardiovascular disease and some cancers. Both fatigue and burnout can erode staff satisfaction and morale and contribute to absenteeism and diminished productivity.

Effects to the patient can also be severe. Tired, fatigued, and burned-out health care workers have slower reaction times, have trouble concentrating, and are more likely to make mistakes. They can overlook significant patient issues or fail to respond to situations that warrant response.

Strategies for Addressing Health Care Worker Fatigue provides an in-depth look at the concepts of worker fatigue and burnout, helps identify those at risk for fatigue and burnout, and provides strategies that organizations can use to reduce the negative effects of these issues.

Chapter One, "Causes and Effects of Fatigue," takes a broad look at the issue of worker fatigue, building awareness of the problem and its consequences.

Chapter Two, "Strategies for Addressing Worker Fatigue," provides real-world solutions to the problems of worker fatigue and sleep deprivation and includes case studies that show how several organizations have addressed these issues.

Chapter Three, "Improving Communication to Help Prevent Fatigue-Related Errors," discusses the importance of effective communication in overcoming any unintended consequences associated with strategies to address worker fatigue.

Chapter Four, "Preventing Worker Burnout," takes a close look at the concept of burnout and how it relates to stress and fatigue. This chapter also provides some ideas about how to address burnout and prevent its negative consequences.

Appendix One provides a suggested readings list that includes articles, Web sites, and other resources that might prove useful when addressing the issues of worker fatigue and burnout.

Appendix Two and Three provide in-depth studies related to health care worker fatigue.

The effective provision of care can occur only when staff members are appropriately prepared to provide that care; if a staff member is fatigued, sleep deprived, or burned out, he or she is not able to provide the best possible care. Consequently, ensuring that workers are not fatigued, chronically sleep deprived, or burned out can contribute to a safe environment for patients and can result in the provision of high-quality care.

Not only is addressing fatigue and burnout good for patients, it is also good for staff. Efforts to address fatigue and burnout can communicate that the organization values its employees, their well-being, and their health. These efforts can help establish a positive and supportive work environment, thus improving staff morale and performance.

Acknowledgements

Joint Commission Resources gratefully acknowledges those who helped in the research and publication of this book, including the following:

- Mark Rosekind, Ph.D., president of Alertness Solutions, Cupertino, California
- Vineet Arora, M.D., associate program director for the internal medicine residency at University of Chicago Hospitals, Chicago
- Steven K. Howard, M.D., director of the Patient Safety Center of Inquiry for VA Palo Alto Health Care System, Palo Alto, California

Thanks especially to Kathleen Vega for her exceptional writing talents.

CHAPTER ONE

Causes and Effects of Fatigue

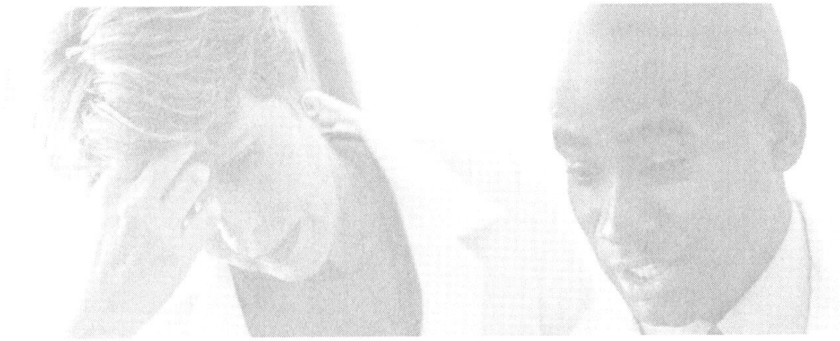

Each year, millions of Americans progress through life tired. Nearly 40% of the workforce in this country experiences fatigue on the job,[1] and nearly 70% of the American public does not get enough sleep during the week.[2]

In the often fast-paced world of health care, worker fatigue has always been a potential patient and provider safety risk. Fatigue has been linked to decreases in performance and increases in medical errors and workplace accidents.

Managing the effects of fatigue and sleep deprivation among health care workers has increased in importance during the past several years, as many health care organizations are dealing with staffing shortages and economic pressures that necessitate extended work shifts and mandatory overtime and often cause worker fatigue.[3] Cost-cutting measures have often led to reductions in staff and created situations in which fewer workers were required to do more.

Today's health care environment requires workers to care for patients who are more acutely ill during their hospital stays. In addition, workers must keep current with rapidly changing technology and treatment options and follow systems and processes that have been put in place to help prevent or mitigate the effects of errors.[3] All these factors combine to create an environment where staff are working harder and longer to address more complex and challenging situations. To effectively treat patients, health care staff members must be alert and focused; however, their schedules are designed to promote exhaustion and fatigue.

Causes of Fatigue

Fatigue is not easily described, and it is defined in many different ways. It can range from a generalized feeling of tiredness and exhaustion to an inability to respond to stimulation. Overall, fatigue is the decreased ability to function due to a lack of energy, a sense of tiredness, or an exhaustion that limits an individual's ability to perform his or her usual functions.[4]

Fatigue is caused by a combination of factors, including the following:

- Insufficient or disrupted sleep
- Poor sleep habits
- Continuous mental or physical activity
- Nonstandard work schedules that lead to disruptions in circadian rhythms
- Multiple jobs, causing both mental and physical weariness
- Multiple caregiving roles outside the work environment (*see* Sidebar 1-1 on page 3)
- Lack of exercise
- Worry or boredom
- Illness
- Abuse of alcohol or other drugs

Fatigue can be acute or chronic. Signs of fatigue can include the following:

- Emotional outbursts, including weepiness
- Irritability
- Excessive giddiness
- Reduced alertness
- Clumsiness
- Weariness
- Lack of motivation
- Exhaustion
- Loss of appetite and digestive problems[4,7]

The Importance of Sleep in Reducing Fatigue

One of the main causes of fatigue is lack of healthy sleep. Although sleep is a biological necessity, like food and water, many people see it as an option rather than a requirement.[8] When managing a busy schedule, individuals often sacrifice healthy sleep to get more done.

It is generally accepted that the average adult needs between six and eight hours of sleep nightly, and yet nearly 70% of Americans sleep less than eight hours each weeknight.[2] People who participate in shift work (*see* page 4) average two to four hours less than this amount.[8]

The Biology of Sleep

A person's sleeping and waking activities are governed in large part by a circadian rhythm, a type of innate biological clock that dictates sleep and wake cycles, daily

Sidebar 1-1. Multiple Caregiving Roles Affect Fatigue

For most health care providers, their jobs are only one aspect of their busy lives. In many cases, health care workers have small children at home and/or are caring for aging parents or other relatives. These multiple caregiving roles can increase fatigue. Combining family caregiving with employment is often difficult because of role conflicts and competing needs.[5] Individuals with multiple caregiving roles frequently sacrifice their own personal or leisure time to fulfill their various commitments. In addition, these individuals sacrifice their own sleep to meet others' needs. For example, staff members might wake at 5 A.M. and work from 7 A.M. to 7 P.M. By the time they arrive home, it is after 8 P.M., and they must perform their evening routines, which might include preparing and eating dinner, helping children with homework, paying bills, doing laundry, and engaging in other household duties. If there is an elderly relative at home, they might have to care for that individual as well. Often with less than seven to eight hours of sleep, they repeat the same routine the next day.[6]

Constant work and caregiving demands with little or no break can generate physical and mental fatigue, which can affect both performance and productivity.[5] One study showed that one-quarter of nurses caring for elderly relatives obtained 5.75 hours or less of sleep on workdays. These nurses were almost 2.5 times more likely than others to make errors at work.[5]

In addition to experiencing significant mental and physical demands due to having multiple caregiving roles, many care providers experience a financial strain because of the economic burden of caring for dependent children and older adults. Therefore, these individuals can be more likely to work additional hours to help pay the bills.[5] All this together results in fatigued and stressed-out individuals who are are at increased risk of making mistakes working extra shifts to make ends meet.

digestive activity, hormone secretions, alertness, and performance levels.[9] In healthy people, this clock cycles approximately every 24 hours and preprograms people to sleep during nighttime hours. People with a normal circadian rhythm have an intense drive for sleep in the evenings and a lesser drive for sleep in the middle of the day.[10]

Within the circadian cycle, the body releases the hormone melatonin. Melatonin, which is secreted by the pineal gland only during times of environmental darkness, causes drowsiness. The hormone cortisol is also released within the circadian cycle, predominantly during the morning. Cortisol, which helps with day waking, regulates metabolism and is released in response to stress.[10]

In conjunction with hormone release, individuals often experience a temperature

> **More Information: The Stages of Sleep**
>
> There are five stages of sleep through which every individual passes. During a healthy sleep episode, individuals cycle through these five stages four times. In the first stage, individuals transition from wakefulness to sleep. It is the lightest stage and the one in which the individual feels drowsy. Light sleep is also a component of stage 2 sleep, which occupies the longest part of a full sleep cycle. Stages 3 and 4 are associated with deep sleep, and it is difficult to arouse a person from stage 3 or stage 4 sleep. During these stages, the body attempts to repair and restore itself through hormone secretion and a lowering of physiologic processes, such as heart rate, blood pressure, and temperature. Rapid eye movement (REM) sleep—the fifth stage—is where dreaming occurs. In this stage, an individual experiences an increase in metabolic processes. Specific characteristics of REM sleep include an electroencephalogram (EEG) pattern similar to that of wakefulness, an irregular pulse, irregular respiration, increased oxygen consumption, increased cerebral blood flow, increased blood pressure, loss of facial muscle tone, and the absence of spinal reflexes.[8]

peak in the late afternoon or early evening and a temperature low in the early morning. There is a correlation between temperature and sleep in that if a person begins sleeping at about the time of the temperature peak rather than at the temperature low, sleep times almost double.[10]

Environmental cues, such as light, outside temperature, and mealtimes, as well as social cues often correspond with an individual's circadian rhythm and prompt people to feel the need for sleep at roughly the same time each night.[8]

Many studies have shown that night sleep is the most restful and restorative type of sleep.[10] Daytime sleep tends to be less productive and lasts for shorter periods of time. For most people, maximum sleepiness occurs between 2 A.M. and 5 A.M. and maximal alertness occurs between noon and 8 P.M.[8]

During sleep, an individual's heart rate, respiratory rate, blood pressure, and metabolic rate are lowered, and brain activity is depressed. Muscle tone and reflexes are also depressed.[10]

The Effects of Shift Work on Worker Fatigue

Hospitals function around the clock and therefore require shift work. Typically, shift work is performed outside the daytime hours of 7 A.M. to 6 P.M. and includes evening shifts, night shifts, rotating shifts, and on-call shifts. More than 20% of the U.S. workforce participates in shift work, and approximately 30% of nurses employed in full-time health care engage in this type of work.[8]

Shift work has many benefits, including higher salaries because of the constantly changing schedule and greater flexibility when coordinating with family schedules and child care.[8] Consequently, it can be an attractive type of work for people who are facing financial issues or who have multiple caregiving roles. Many health care workers who engage in shift work, including interns, physicians, and nurses, are strapped financially and often work second jobs. In some cases, these individuals moonlight in their own organizations to make extra money. (More information on moonlighting can be found in Chapter Two.)

In health care, individuals who participate in shift work or who engage in prolonged work hours—such as shifts lasting 12 hours or more—are more likely to be fatigued than those who work a more regular schedule. Evening and night shift workers can be particularly susceptible to fatigue. As previously mentioned, human beings are biologically wired to be awake during the day and asleep at night. Work schedules that oppose this natural rhythm can generate physiologic disruptions that lead to significantly degraded performance and increased risks to health and safety.[11]

Night workers must work during the nocturnal release of melatonin and sleep during the day without it, and they must also work against the cortisol-induced desire for morning wakefulness.[10] This can result in difficulty falling asleep during the day and difficulty staying awake at night. It also results in short sleep periods during the day, leading to a reduced amount of sleep. Consequently, fatigue accumulates faster during night work

More Information: Sleeping Patterns While on Call

Several studies have looked at the sleeping patterns of health care workers while they are on call. One study showed that surgical residents averaged 5 to 6 hours of sleep while on call. Another study showed that nearly 90% of obstetrics/gynecology (OB/GYN) residents reported less than 4 hours of sleep while on call, and a group of anesthesiologists reported an average of 4.8 hours of sleep while on call. Still another study showed that residents' daytime sleepiness was near or below levels associated with clinical sleep disorders.[12]

More Information: Shift Work More Difficult with Age

The ability to successfully navigate shift work has been linked to age. An individual's ability to adjust his or her circadian rhythm decreases with age, as does his or her ability to achieve sleep that is uninterrupted and of sufficient length. Once an individual reaches 40 to 50 years of age, there is a natural tendency to perform better and be more alert in the morning. Consequently, older staff members can have difficulty adjusting to evening, night, and rotating shifts.[10]

More Information: Consistent Night Shift Work Might Be Preferable

Staff members who work permanently—or at least for long, continuous periods—on the night shift might be less likely to suffer sleep deprivation effects than those whose shifts are continuously changing. It is hypothesized that this is because the body is able to adjust its sleep cycle, given enough time.[10] Consequently, slower rotations of two to three weeks or fixed rotations can help prevent some of the problems associated with shift work.

than during day work.[10] When an individual is deprived of sleep, the natural circadian rhythm is disrupted, and the person craves that lost sleep.[10]

Of all the types of shift work, rotating shifts might have the most impact on worker fatigue. Changes in work schedules from days to nights and from nights to days are often too rapid to allow an individual's circadian rhythm to adapt. This places many providers in a permanent state of "jet lag," as they attempt to remain awake at work and asleep at home.[13]

The direction of shift work also plays a role in worker fatigue. For workers who change from one shift to another, a forward rotation from morning shifts to evening shifts is easier to tolerate physiologically because the natural circadian rhythm tends to move forward.

In addition to shift work, extended work hours can also cause worker fatigue. With the nationwide nursing shortage, many organizations are routinely asking, or in some cases requiring, staff members to work longer hours or extra shifts. Nurses, in particular, tend to work longer than their scheduled shifts on a regular basis. A recent study showed that hospital staff nurses who work longer than scheduled on a daily basis average an additional 55 minutes longer than scheduled each day. Overtime hours were involved in 85% of the shifts scheduled for 8 hours, 79% of the shifts scheduled for 8 to 12 hours, and 78% of shifts scheduled for 12 hours or more.[5] One complication associated with unscheduled overtime is that workers might not be able to plan ahead for such overtime and might not get sufficient sleep, and thus they might begin their shift with a sleep deficit.

The Consequences of Worker Fatigue

Fatigue can affect an individual's performance and personality in a variety of ways, including the following:

- Reduce decision-making ability
- Prolong response time
- Increase lapses in attention
- Negatively affect short-term memory and recall

- Impair data-processing ability
- Reduce attention to detail
- Impair concentration
- Compromise problem-solving ability
- Affect speech
- Reduce motivation
- Increase feelings of anger and anxiety
- Decrease vigor and positive feelings, such as happiness
- Increase irritability, moodiness, and depression
- Decrease ability to communicate[14-15]
- Create problems associated with a disruption in family life
- Isolate individuals from family, friends, and social activities

Lack of sleep can especially affect performance. For example, after one night of missed sleep, cognitive performance can decrease 25%. After a second night of missed sleep, cognitive performance can decrease 40%.[16] One landmark study found that after 17 hours of sustained wakefulness, cognitive performance among test subjects decreased to a level equivalent to that of a person with a blood alcohol concentration (BAC) of 0.05%. A BAC of 0.08% is the legal standard for intoxication in most states. After 24 hours of sustained wakefulness, performance decreased to a level equivalent to that of a person with a BAC of roughly 0.10%.[17]

More Information: Shift Work Sleep Disorder

Shift work is not appropriate for everyone. Some individuals are unable to adapt their circadian rhythms to shift work and can, over time, experience severe health problems. In minor cases, individuals experience a general malaise, headache, insomnia, or a need to sleep at every opportunity. In more serious cases, individuals develop a shift work sleep disorder in which they experience a constant or recurring pattern of sleep interruption that results in insomnia during the day and excessive sleepiness during night work. An estimated 10% of the 6 million regular night shift workers in the United States have been diagnosed with this disorder. This disorder can affect an individual's quality of life as well as his or her ability to function at work.[8]

Effects of Fatigue on Patient Safety

Physicians and nurses need focused attention, sound judgment, quick reaction time, and clear reasoning to perform their jobs accurately, adequately, and efficiently. Whether administering an intravenous (IV) medication or monitoring a patient during anesthesia administration, degradation of attention, memory, and coordination due to fatigue can affect a performance; affect patient safety; and lead to adverse events.[16] Fatigue can affect physicians' and nurses' technical skills and their ability to perform specific procedures. For example, studies have shown that surgeons have less surgical dexterity and operate more slowly when fatigued.[15]

More Information: Addressing Sleep Debt

Sleep loss over several days, weeks, and months leads to sleep debt, which is the cumulative effect of lost sleep. Although most healthy people can function relatively well even after 3 or 4 days of inadequate sleep, problems occur when a sleep debt is not repaid. An issue with many health care schedules—including 12-hour shifts, night shifts, and on-call shifts—is that sleep debt accumulates across several days of insufficient sleep, and if an individual does not have adequate time to make up the debt, a chronic level of fatigue develops.[3]

A sleep debt cannot be repaid immediately. In other words, 1 good night's sleep after 5 nights of poor sleep will not balance the scale. If an individual sleeps less than 5 or 6 hours across 7 nights, the sleep debt is approximately 15 to 20 hours. At least 48 hours off duty is needed to recover this sleep deficit.[18]

Physicians-in-training who work traditional schedules with recurrent 24-hour shifts have a greatly increased risk of injuring their patients or others and incur the following additional risks compared to those whose scheduled work is limited to 15 consecutive hours:

- They make 36% more serious medical errors.
- They make five times as many serious diagnostic errors.
- They have twice as many on-the-job attention failures at night.
- They suffer 61% more needlestick and other sharps injuries after 20 consecutive hours of work.
- They report making 300% more fatigue-related medical errors that lead to patient death.[13] (For more on this study, see Appendix Two on page 113.)

Nurses encounter similar fatigue-related risks. A study of nurses showed that the risk of a nurse making an error significantly increased when the nurse's work shift exceeded 12 hours, when overtime was worked, or when work hours exceeded 40 per week. In fact, the likelihood of a nurse making an error was three times higher when the shift lasted 12.5 hours or more. This study also indicated that many nurses worked beyond their scheduled shift times, and those individuals who did work beyond their 12-hour shifts were most vulnerable to making errors.[19]

Mistakes caused by fatigued individuals are most likely to occur during routine tasks and tasks that require sustained concentration. Effects on urgent tasks or those that require short yet significant bursts of mental energy are less severe. Interestingly, fatigue causes fewer performance problems in workers with more control over their work because they can schedule non-urgent tasks or tasks that require sustained concentration for times when they are at their best. Physicians can thus cope better with fatigue than staff members who have less job flexibility, such as nurses.[18]

In addition to increasing the risk of medical error, fatigue can contribute to feelings of depression, anger, and resentment in health care workers, which can lead to a sense of detachment and a lack of compassion for patients.[20] One study of residents revealed that the subjects were often inattentive and abrupt with patients and family members because of fatigue. Many of the subjects interviewed described a noticeable loss of empathy, compassion, and concern for their patients because of fatigue. When fatigued, the residents experienced an urge to objectify patients and move them through the system rather than care for the patients as individuals and focus on their needs.[21] When care providers are fatigued and experience diminished compassion, potential lapses in patient safety can occur, including patient complaints being dismissed, potential health issues being overlooked, and serious health problems not being recognized.

Effects of Fatigue on Provider Safety

Patients are not the only ones affected by fatigued health care workers; the workers themselves experience detrimental effects of chronic fatigue. Physical and mental health, interpersonal relationships, and the ability to perform the tasks of daily life can all be affected by acute sleep loss and fatigue. Highly fatigued individuals are at an increased risk of getting sick due to diminished immune response and other related factors. According to a recent study in *HR News*, fatigued workers

More Information: Microsleeps

Ongoing sleep loss can lead to microsleeps. These occur when individuals fall asleep for very brief periods at inappropriate times. Sometimes these sleeps can occur when performing tasks, such as during surgery, when driving an automobile, or when talking with a patient or his or her family. Microsleeps last only a few seconds, are completely involuntary, and occur without the individual realizing he or she is falling asleep. During a microsleep, the individual is incapable of paying attention, is unresponsive to external stimuli, and therefore is completely unable to perform safely and efficiently.[3] The more sleep deprived an individual is, the more frequently microsleeps are likely to occur.

More Information: Types of Errors Caused by Fatigue

Often, fatigue-related mistakes involve failure to recognize the existence of a serious problem. For example, giving the wrong antibiotic to a septic patient is not typically a fatigue-related mistake; however, failing to recognize and diagnose a septic patient is a typical fatigue-related error.[18]

More Information: Drowsy Driving

Fatigue, specifically fatigue caused by sleepiness, and driving is a dangerous combination. This combination can be just as risky and just as fatal as drinking and driving. As previously mentioned, sleepiness and fatigue can slow reaction time, decrease awareness, impair judgment, and increase an individual's risk of crashing. In some cases, microsleeps can occur while driving, causing a complete loss of focus and concentration on the road and an inability to respond to environmental stimuli. In a recent study, more than 40% of health care workers reported nodding off while driving, and 39% reported near misses or accidents, caused by being tired.[11]

In addition to the physical dangers of driving while fatigued, several states are considering legislation that would allow police to charge drowsy drivers with criminal negligence if they injure or kill someone while driving if they have not had adequate sleep.[25] By placing employees in a situation where they are forced to drive drowsy, organizations are placing them at risk not only for bodily harm but also potential criminal charges. In the future, such litigation could be tied back to the organization in which the drowsy driver works, as the organization is responsible for setting the individual's schedule.

cost U.S. employers $136.4 billion annually in health-related lost productivity.[7]

Shift workers in particular can suffer ill effects from fatigue. For example, shift workers are more likely than others to struggle with obesity, cardiovascular diseases, and gastrointestinal disorders such as peptic ulcers, indigestion, diarrhea, and constipation, in part because of disruptions in their circadian rhythms and also because they might consume more high-fat, high-sodium fast foods and get less exercise than non-shift workers.[10] Increased risk for irregular menstrual cycles, premature labor, and miscarriage is also seen in shift workers,[10] as is increased risk of certain cancers, including breast cancer, as compared with non-shift workers.[13]

In addition to the detrimental health effects, there is a well-documented connection between long work hours, night shifts, and an increased likelihood of on-the-job accidents.[3] Such accidents can include needlestick injuries and bloodborne pathogen exposure. One recent study found that the number of hours worked per day, the number of weekends worked per month, and whether individuals worked evening and night shifts were significantly associated with needlestick injuries.[22]

Fatigue is not a contributor only to workplace accidents but also to accidents that occur outside the workplace. One study found that first-year medical interns who worked shifts longer than 24 hours were more than twice as likely as interns who worked shorter shifts to be in car crashes after leaving work and five times as likely to have near misses.[23] Studies also report increased rates of crashes in nurses when driving home after working night shifts.[24]

Working in Denial

Many health care workers are not aware that working long hours can affect performance, or they feel they are immune to the risks associated with fatigue and sleep deprivation. Despite lack of sleep and feelings of fatigue, health care providers fully expect to be able to perform reliably with high levels of precision and accuracy. They deny the impact of fatigue on their performance even though they have experienced the negative effects firsthand.[6] Consider the story of an OB/GYN resident who was working the 35th hour of his 36-hour shift. He was examining a 28-year-old woman who had delivered a baby earlier in the evening. In reviewing her chart, the resident was unable to understand the notes of the previous on-call resident and was irritated at the previous physician's incoherent ramblings. To help clarify the information in the chart, the resident began asking the woman questions about her delivery. The woman indicated that she answered those questions before for him, when he visited her 3 hours earlier. In looking closely at the notes and at the patient, the resident realized he had taken the previous notes and actually examined this woman several hours before but had no recollection of her or her case. These types of stories are not uncommon among physicians and nurses, as they often progress through their shifts in fog-like states.

Although evidence shows that fatigue and sleep deprivation can negatively affect performance, it is a common perception that health care workers can be trained to function for long periods with no rest. In fact, some people feel that long, grueling work schedules are not only not a problem but are a benefit because such shifts help health care workers prepare for emergency situations. The irony of this is that sleep deprivation in no way helps performance, and, in fact, workers who are adequately rested are more likely to be able to work unusually long hours when an emergency requires it. Willingness to work extra shifts and longer hours is often perceived as "professional"; however, the need for sleep is a human physiological process, and a commitment to stay awake cannot overcome the drive for sleep.[18]

There is another common perception that the amount of learning required for medical students and residents is so great that sleep must be sacrificed. However, sleep deprivation negatively affects a person's ability to retain information, and keeping residents up for long periods of time can consequently be detrimental to their education.

Legislation Associated with Fatigue

Fatigue and its effects on health care workers are not just concerns of health care organizations. Legislators at federal and state levels, as well as accrediting agencies, patient safety groups, professional associations, and the public, are all becoming increasingly aware of the effects of fatigue in health care. In response to this concern, Congress and several state legislatures have introduced bills to reduce the number of hours worked by medical residents and nurses and to set mandatory staffing ratios.

The movement toward reforming the number of hours worked by hospital residents can be traced back to a highly publicized 1984 court case involving the death of Libby Zion, an 18-year-old college student. When Ms. Zion was admitted to a New York hospital, she had a fever, was flailing her arms and legs, and had flu-like symptoms. A resident who had been on duty for more than 19 hours ordered a drug that interacted with a prescription the patient was taking. Ms. Zion died 8 hours after admission. Her death was blamed in part on a system that keeps residents chronically exhausted. Although the verdict on this case was mixed, Sydney Zion—Libby's father and a former federal prosecutor—was successful in making teaching hospitals more accountable for the supervision of medical residents and interns.[3] This case galvanized public support for limiting resident work hours.

The Accreditation Council for Graduate Medical Education's Work in Limiting Duty Hours

In 2003, the Accreditation Council for Graduate Medical Education (ACGME) (*see* Sidebar 1-2 on page 13) issued revised standards for medical resident duty hours. These standards, which were updated in July 2007, require organizations to limit resident duty hours to 80 hours per week, averaged over a 4-week period, inclusive of all in-house call activities. Residents must be provided with 1 day in 7 free from all educational and clinical responsibilities and be allowed adequate time for rest and personal activities. (For a complete listing of the ACGME guidelines, *see* Figure 1-1 on page 14.)

These guidelines stemmed from the fact that medical residents were working extreme hours, sometimes 120 hours per week, leaving only 48 hours for family, personal life, and sleep. Although some consider these standards stringent, they are more lenient than those of other industries with similar fatigue-related hazards, such as the commercial airline industry.[3]

Organizations that do not comply with the ACGME's standards face adverse action, including probation and withdrawal of accreditation. Loss of ACGME accreditation results in lack of eligibility for Medicare graduate medical education funding. In addition, medical residents in a program that has lost ACGME accreditation may lose their eligibility to take board certification examinations.[3]

Organizations have responded to the ACGME regulations in a variety of ways.

Some have extended rotations to allow individuals to recover their sleep debts between rotations, whereas others have implemented fixed night shifts. In many cases, organizations have had to hire additional staff and clinicians. For example, organizations have hired nocturnists—internists who work a fixed schedule at night—or additional shift staff. More information on complying with ACGME duty hour guidelines can be found in Chapter Two.

The Government's Role in Addressing Worker Fatigue

As previously mentioned, both the federal and state governments have gotten involved in the issue of worker fatigue. In January 2007, Nevada Congressman Harry Reid introduced S73, a bill that amended the Social Security Act to provide for patient protection by establishing minimum nurse staffing ratios at certain Medicare providers. Although this bill addresses staffing issues, it also acknowledges the fact that because of these staffing issues, registered nurses are being required to perform work under conditions that do not support quality health care or a healthful work environment. (For more information on the bill and its requirements, go to http://thomas.loc.gov.)

Many state legislatures are addressing the issue of worker fatigue by considering or enacting legislation restricting mandatory overtime for nurses and other health care professionals.[3] (*See* Sidebar 1-3, at right.) In addition, the Institute of

Sidebar 1-2. Accreditation Council for Graduate Medical Education (ACGME)

The ACGME is responsible for the accreditation of more than 7,900 resident physician medical training programs within the United States.[3] Accreditation is accomplished through a peer review process and is based on established standards and guidelines. The aim of these standards and guidelines is to promote safe patient care, resident learning, and resident well-being.[27]

Sidebar 1-3. States Addressing the Issue of Mandatory Overtime[30]

California
Colorado
Connecticut
Florida
Hawaii
Illinois
Iowa
Kentucky
Maine
Maryland
Massachusetts
Minnesota
Missouri
New Jersey
New York
Ohio
Oregon
Pennsylvania
Rhode Island
Virginia
Washington
West Virginia
Wisconsin

Figure 1-1.
Accreditation Council for Graduate Medical Education (ACGME) Resident Duty Hours

Duty Hours Language

VI. Resident Duty Hours in the Learning and Working Environment

A. Principles

1. The program must be committed to and be responsible for promoting patient safety and resident well-being and to providing a supportive educational environment.
2. The learning objectives of the program must not be compromised by excessive reliance on residents to fulfill service obligations.
3. Didactic and clinical education must have priority in the allotment of residents' time and energy.
4. Duty hour assignments must recognize that faculty and residents collectively have responsibility for the safety and welfare of patients.

B. Supervision of Residents

The program must ensure that qualified faculty provides appropriate supervision of residents in patient care activities.

C. Fatigue

Faculty and residents must be educated to recognize the signs of fatigue and sleep deprivation and must adopt and apply policies to prevent and counteract its potential negative effects on patient care and learning.

D. Duty Hours ***(the terms in this section are defined in the ACGME Glossary and apply to all programs)***

Duty hours are defined as all clinical and academic activities related to the program; i.e., patient care (both inpatient and outpatient), administrative duties relative to patient care, the provision for transfer of patient care, time spent in-house during call activities, and scheduled activities, such as conferences. Duty hours do not include reading and preparation time spent away from the duty site.

1. Duty hours must be limited to 80 hours per week, averaged over a four-week period, inclusive of all in-house call activities.

Figure 1-1. (continued)
Accreditation Council for Graduate Medical Education (ACGME) Resident Duty Hours

2. Residents must be provided with one day in seven free from all educational and clinical responsibilities, averaged over a four-week period, inclusive of call.
3. Adequate time for rest and personal activities must be provided. This should consist of a 10-hour time period provided between all daily duty periods and after in-house call.

E. On-call Activities

1. In-house call must occur no more frequently than every third night, averaged over a four-week period.
2. Continuous on-site duty, including in-house call, must not exceed 24 consecutive hours. Residents may remain on duty for up to 6 additional hours to participate in didactic activities, transfer care of patients, conduct outpatient clinics, and maintain continuity of medical and surgical care.
3. No new patients may be accepted after 24 hours of continuous duty.
4. At-home call (or pager call)
   a) The frequency of at-home call is not subject to the every-third-night, or 24+6 limitation. However, at-home call must not be so frequent as to preclude rest and reasonable personal time for each resident.
   b) Residents taking at-home call must be provided with one day in seven completely free from all educational and clinical responsibilities, averaged over a four-week period.
   c) When residents are called into the hospital from home, the hours residents spend in-house are counted toward the 80-hour limit.

F. Moonlighting

1. Moonlighting must not interfere with the ability of the resident to achieve the goals and objectives of the educational program.
2. Internal moonlighting must be considered part of the 80-hour weekly limit on duty hours.

(continued)

Figure 1-1. (continued)
Accreditation Council for Graduate Medical Education (ACGME) Resident Duty Hours

G. Duty Hours Exceptions

A Review Committee may grant exceptions for up to 10% or a maximum of 88 hours to individual programs based on a sound educational rationale.

1. In preparing a request for an exception, the program director must follow the duty hour exception policy from the ACGME Manual on Policies and Procedures.
2. Prior to submitting the request to the Review Committee, the program director must obtain approval of the institution's GMEC and DIO.

***

ACGME Approved: February 13, 2007
Effective: July 1, 2007
For more information on the ACGME requirements, go to www.acgme.org.

Source: Accreditation Council for Graduate Medical Education (ACGME), Chicago. Used with permission.

On July 1, 2003, a new common ACGME standard for resident duty hours went into effect. Above is the language of this requirement.

Medicine's Board of Health Care Services has recommended that state regulatory bodies prohibit nursing staff from providing patient care in any combination of scheduled shifts, mandatory overtime, or voluntary overtime in excess of 12 hours in any given 24-hour period and in excess of 60 hours per 7-day period.[29]

Mandatory overtime is a controversial and potentially dangerous practice that occurs when an individual, such as a nurse, is told that he or she could be fired, subjected to disciplinary proceedings, or lose his or her license if he or she refuses to stay beyond the regularly scheduled shift or come to work on his or her day off. In some cases, mandatory overtime is more subtle; individuals are not actually threatened with job loss or disciplinary action but feel there will be repercussions if they refuse to work extra hours.[19] Mandatory overtime is an issue in many health care organizations. In 2004, one survey indicated that more than one-quarter of participants reported working mandatory overtime at least once during the data-gathering period.[19]

Joint Commission Requirements

The Joint Commission standards require organizations to manage their safety risks, including risks that affect the safety and health of patients, staff, and other people coming to the hospital. To comply with the standards, organizations should consider addressing the issue of worker fatigue, as it is a safety risk for both patients and staff.

Addressing worker fatigue can help prevent errors, improve staff performance, enhance worker morale, and lead to patient satisfaction and safety. There are many ways to address the issue of worker fatigue; Chapter Two discusses some of these strategies.

References

1. Fatigue in the workplace is common and costly. *Medical News Today*, Jan. 15, 2007. http://www.medicalnewstoday.com/medicalnews.php?newsid=60732 (accessed Dec. 1, 2007).

2. National Sleep Foundation: *2002 "Sleep in America"*, Poll. Mar. 2002. http://www.kintera.org/atf/cf/%7BF6BF2668-A1B4-4FE8-8D1A-A5D39340D9CB%7D/2002SleepInAmericaPoll.pdf (accessed Dec. 1, 2007).

3. Fatigue in healthcare workers. Healthcare Risk Control. Risk Analysis Employment Issues 14 (Suppl. A), *ECRI* Jan. 2006.

4. Smith B: Test your stamina for workplace fatigue. *Nurs Manage* 35:38–40, Oct. 2004.

5. Scott L., Hwang W., Rogers A.: The impact of multiple care giving roles on fatigue, stress, and work performance among hospital staff nurses. *J Nurs Adm* 36:86–95, Feb. 2006.

6. Beyea S.: Too tired to work safely. *AORN J* 80:559–560, Sep. 2004.

7. Gurchiek K.: Study finds eye-opening cost associated with fatigued workers. *HR News*, Jan. 30, 2007.

8. Blachowicz E., Letizia M.: The challenges of shift work. *Medsurg Nurs* 15:274–280, Oct. 2006.

9. Howard S.K., et al.: Fatigue in anesthesia: Implications and strategies for patient and provider safety. *Anesthesiology* 97:1281–1294, 2002.

10. Muecke S.: Effects of rotating night shifts: A literature review. *J Adv Nurs* 30:433–439, 2005.

11. Rosekind M.: Managing work schedules: An alertness and safety perspective. In Kryger M., Roth T., Dement W. (eds.): *Principles and Practice of Sleep Medicine*. Philadelphia: Elsevier Science, 2005, pp. 680–690.

12. Howard S., et al.: The risks and implications of excessive daytime sleepiness in resident physicians. *Acad Med* 77:1019–1025, Oct. 2002.

13. Lockley S., et al.: Effects of health care provider work hours and sleep deprivation on safety and performance. *Jt Comm J Qual Patient Saf* 33:7–18, Nov. 2007.

14. Poissonnet C.M., Veron M.: Health effects of work schedules in healthcare professions. *J Clin Nurs* 9:13–23, Jan. 2000.

15. Eastridge B.J., et al.: Effects of sleep deprivation on the performance of simulated laparoscopic surgical skill. *Am J Surg* 186:169–174, Aug. 2003.

16. Jha A., Duncan B., Bates D.: Fatigue, Sleepiness and Medical Errors. In Shojania K.G., et al. (eds.): *Making Health Care Safer: A Critical Analysis of Patient Safety Practices.* Rockville, MD: Agency for Healthcare Research and Quality, 2001, pp. 519–532.

17. Dawson D., et al.: Fatigue, alcohol, and performance impairment. *Nature* 388:235, Jul. 17, 1997.

18. Olson L., Ambrogetti A.: Working harder—Working dangerously? Fatigue and performance in hospitals. *Med J Aust* 168:614–616, 1998.

19. Rogers A.E., et al.: The working hours of hospital staff nurses and patient safety. *Health Aff (Millwood)* 23:202–212, Jul.–Aug. 2004.

20. Gaba D.M., Howard S.K.: Patient safety: Fatigue among clinicians and the safety of patients. *N Engl J Med* 17:129–55, Oct. 17, 2002.

21. Papp K., et al.: The effects of sleep loss and fatigue on resident-physicians: A multi-institutional, mixed-method study. *Acad Med* 79:394–406, May 2004.

22. Trinkoff A.M., et al.: Work schedule, needle use, and needlestick injuries among registered nurses. *Infect Control Hosp Epidemiol* 28:156–164, Feb. 2007.

23. Barger L.K., et al.: Extended work shifts and the risk of motor vehicle crashes among interns. *N Engl J Me*d 13:125–134, Jan. 13, 2005.

24. Caruso C., Condon M.: Night shifts and fatigue: Coping skills for the working nurse. *Am J Nurs* 106:88, Aug. 2006.

25. National Sleep Foundation: *What Is Drowsy Driving?* http://www.drowsydriving.org/site/c.lqLPIROCKtF/b.3468651/k.7145/What_is_Drowsy_Driving.htm (accessed Dec. 2, 2007).

26. Fields H.: Wake up, doc. *U.S. News & World Report,* Dec. 8, 2003.

27. American Council for Graduate Medical Education home page. http://www.acgme.org (accessed Dec. 10, 2007).

28. Accreditation Council for Graduate Medical Education: *Duty Hours Language.*, Jul. 1, 2007. http://www.acgme.org/acWebsite/dutyHours/dh_Lang703.pdf (accessed Dec. 10, 2007).

29. Board Health Care Services, Institute of Medicine of the National Academies: Keeping patients safe: Transforming the work environment of nurses. *Am J Public Health* 82:1011–1014, Jul. 1992.

30. Service Employees International Union: *State Legislation to Limit Mandatory Overtime.* http://www.seiu.org/health/hosp/mandatory_overtime2/mot_factsheet.cfm (accessed Dec. 1, 2007).

CHAPTER TWO

Strategies for Addressing Worker Fatigue

Solving the worker fatigue problem in the U.S. health care system might, on the surface, seem simple: Health care workers, including physicians, nurses, pharmacists, and other staff, must get more sleep. However, achieving this goal can be challenging and requires commitment from health care workers and the organizations in which they work.

Effectively managing fatigue in any setting that operates 24 hours a day, 7 days a week is a complex endeavor, and there is no magic solution that will completely eliminate the problem.[1] Every organization will need to decide what approach works best for it. Most organizations will need to use a combination of strategies, and critically examine culture in which those strategies will be implemented.

One possible way to address worker fatigue and its patient and provider safety consequences is to develop an alertness management program. This term, coined by Mark Rosekind, Ph.D., describes a multifaceted approach that includes education, alertness strategies, scheduling practices, healthy sleep diagnoses, and organizational policy support.[1] Although every organization's alertness management program will look different, the following sections discuss some things to keep in mind when designing such a program.

Providing Education on Fatigue and Its Consequences

Despite the health benefits of a good night's sleep and the health and safety risks of a poor one, many people do not place value on sleeping. As mentioned in Chapter One, sleeping is just as important to achieving a healthy lifestyle as good nutrition and exercise. However, many people feel that they can function adequately on little sleep and might even feel that they perform better. In the health care arena, many health care workers see sleep deprivation and the fatigue that results from it as a necessary part of the job.

Education should be the foundation for any effort to reduce fatigue in the work setting. Although organizations might rework schedules to provide opportunities for health care workers to get more rest, there is no guarantee that a health care worker will use that nonwork time to sleep. It is imperative that health care workers receive comprehensive education on fatigue and sleep deprivation and the risks associated with them. This education can help prompt individuals to use their time off to get the sleep they need.

All staff members in an organization who work irregular shifts—including nurses, technicians, pharmacists, maintenance personnel, residents, and physicians—should receive education on sleep deprivation and fatigue because everyone can benefit from healthy sleep and reduced fatigue. Following is some information organizations should consider including in an education program on sleep and fatigue:

- How sleep works
- Sleep deprivation and sleep debt
- Microsleeps and their consequences
- The effects of sleep deprivation and fatigue on performance
- The patient and provider risks associated with sleep deprivation and fatigue
- Good sleep habits
- Signs of fatigue, including irritability, slowed physical and mental reactions, forgetfulness, and an inability to focus
- Available approaches to reduce the risks associated with fatigue
- Sleep disorders and how to recognize their signs and symptoms

Education on sleep deprivation and fatigue can and should take many forms, including lectures, articles in staff newsletters, pocket pieces with important facts, posters in staff break rooms, and conferences or retreats that delve into the topic. Interactive education, including questionnaires that assess an individual's level of fatigue (*see* Figure 2-1 on page 23) or discussions of hypothetical scenarios involving fatigued workers, could be beneficial in helping staff members understand the problems associated with fatigue and ways to combat it.

Education on sleep and fatigue should be ongoing and should relate directly to the experiences of the staff. Integrating fatigue education into an ongoing education program can create the opportunity for this information to become part of the organizational culture.[1]

As with any other type of education, there should be some measure of whether the education is effective. This might take the form of a questionnaire, a brief quiz that tests knowledge, or focus groups that gather opinions about the education at the end of the education session. In addition, observing worker behavior and tracking the

Figure 2-1.
The Epworth Sleepiness Scale

Developed by Murray John, M.D., of Epworth Hospital in Melbourne, Australia, the Epworth Sleepiness Scale is a questionnaire that measures daytime sleepiness.[3] Not only can this questionnaire help show a staff person his or her level of sleepiness, it can also be used to diagnosis a sleep disorder. A score of 10 or more is considered sleepy. A score of 18 or more is very sleepy. If an individual's score is 10 or more on this test, that person should consider whether he or she is obtaining adequate sleep, needs to improve his or her sleep hygiene, and/or needs to see a sleep specialist.[4]

Use the following scale to rate your chance of dozing or sleeping:
0 = would *never* doze or sleep
1 = *slight* chance of dozing or sleeping
2 = *moderate* chance of dozing or sleeping
3 = *high* chance of dozing or sleeping

Situation
____ Chance of dozing or sleeping
____ Sitting and reading
____ Watching TV
____ Sitting inactive in a public place
____ Being a passenger in a motor vehicle for an hour or more
____ Lying down in the afternoon
____ Sitting and talking to someone
____ Sitting quietly after lunch (no alcohol)
____ Stopped for a few minutes in traffic while driving
____ **Total score (This is your Epworth score)**

Source: Adapted from University of Maryland Medical Center Sleep Disorders Center: *Sleep-Related Tests & Quizzes: Epworth Sleepiness Scale.* http://www.umm.edu/sleep/epworth_sleep.htm (accessed Dec. 10, 2007).

number of reported incidents that relate to fatigue can help determine the need for further education. (More information about reporting fatigue-related incidents can be found on page 56)

Any education provided on sleep deprivation and fatigue should be supported by the organization's actions. For example, if an organization teaches staff members

More Information: Sleep, Alertness, and Fatigue Education in Residency (SAFER)

One specific tool organizations can use to educate residents about sleep deprivation is the Sleep, Alertness, and Fatigue Education in Residency (SAFER) program, developed by the American Academy of Sleep Medicine. This program, which is used by many teaching hospitals across the country, involves a 60- to 90-minute lecture covering the neurological characteristics of sleeping and waking, the effects of sleep loss on the personal and professional lives of residents, and effective strategies to reduce fatigue and improve performance.[2] Although this program can be effective, organizations should not rely on it solely to improve the sleep habits of residents. Education on sleep and fatigue can take many forms, and merely lecturing staff once on the importance of sleep will not change habits.

that it is important to get more sleep and come to the job well rested, then schedules for employees must allow time to achieve those goals. If the culture and actions of the organization do not support healthy sleep, then education on the topic will not be effective. (More information on creating a culture that supports fatigue-reducing strategies can be found on page 28.)

Using Alertness Strategies to Overcome Fatigue

In addition to education, another component of an effective alertness management program is alertness strategies; these are specific activities that health care workers can engage in to help combat the effects of fatigue. Workers should be educated on common alertness strategies, and organization policy should support and encourage the use of these strategies. The following sections discuss some of the most common strategies.

Caffeine

Caffeine is sometimes called the world's most popular drug, and, in moderation, it can be helpful in reducing the effects of fatigue. Although it does not address the underlying reasons behind fatigue, the use of caffeine can help combat the effects of fatigue, at least temporarily.

Although caffeine cannot replace sleep, it can temporarily make an individual feel more alert by blocking sleep-inducing chemicals in the brain and increasing adrenaline production.[7] For staff members to use caffeine effectively, they should understand how and when to use it and for how long it will be beneficial. Staff should know what dose is needed to enhance alertness and mental functioning, how much caffeine is contained in different drinks and food, and what is the best

More Information: Educating Staff on Good Sleep Habits

Although organizations can do a lot to help ensure that health care workers get healthy sleep, some of the responsibility for sleep falls to the individual. For this reason, it is important to educate staff on healthy sleep habits and encourage them to adopt these habits into their daily routines. Some important sleep habits to cover within education sessions include the following.[5]

Go to bed and wake up at a consistent time each day, including on weekends. A regular wake-up time in the morning strengthens the circadian function and can help with sleep onset at night.

Establish a regular bedtime routine. A relaxing routine activity right before bedtime, conducted away from bright lights, helps an individual separate his or her sleep time from activities that can cause excitement, stress, or anxiety. Relaxing activities can include taking a warm bath, reading a book or magazine, and listening to music. Relaxation therapies can also be helpful to avoid tension and stress. Before bedtime, individuals should avoid arousing activities such as working, paying bills, engaging in competitive games, and family problem solving. Individuals trying to go to sleep should avoid exposure to bright light before bed because it signals to the neurons that help control the sleep–wake cycle that it is time to awaken, not to sleep.

Create a sleep-conducive environment. An environment that is conducive to sleep is dark, quiet, comfortable, and cool. To achieve this type of environment, individuals should consider using blackout curtains, eye shades, earplugs, white noise, humidifiers, fans, and other devices.

Sleep on a comfortable mattress and pillows. An individual should make sure his or her mattress is both comfortable and supportive. The life expectancy for a typical mattress is about 9 or 10 years for most good-quality mattresses. Individuals should also try to keep their pillows free of allergens that might affect sleep.

Do not eat or drink right before bed. Eating or drinking too much can make an individual less comfortable when settling down for bed. It is best to avoid heavy meals close to bedtime. Also, spicy foods can cause heartburn, which leads to difficulty falling asleep and discomfort during the night. It is important to try to restrict fluids close to bedtime to prevent nighttime trips to the bathroom, though some people find milk or herbal, noncaffeinated teas to be soothing and a helpful part of a bedtime routine.

(continued)

More Information: Educating Staff on Good Sleep Habits (continued)

Exercise regularly. In general, exercising regularly makes it easier to fall asleep and contributes to sounder sleep. However, exercising sporadically or right before going to bed may make falling asleep more difficult. In addition to making an individual more alert, excersise causes body temperature to rise for as long as six hours. A cooler body temperature is associated with sleep onset.

Avoid caffeine close to bedtime. Caffeine is a stimulant, which means it can produce an alerting effect. Avoiding caffeine within six to eight hours of going to bed can help improve sleep quality.

Avoid nicotine. Nicotine is a stimulant. Smoking before bedtime causes difficultly falling asleep. When smokers go to sleep, they experience withdrawal symptoms from nicotine, which can also cause sleep problems. Nicotine can also cause nightmares and problems waking in the morning.

Avoid alcohol close to bedtime. Although many people think of alcohol as a sedative, it actually disrupts sleep, causing nighttime waking.

To encourage night-shift workers to get good sleep, organizations might also want to give the following suggestions:

- Install opaque coverings over windows and under doorways to prevent light from entering the sleeping space.
- Turn off phones to ensure uninterrupted sleep.
- Use a white noise machine or earplugs to minimize noise disturbances.
- Instruct family members and friends when and when not to wake you.
- Keep the sleeping space cool and use an appropriate amount of covers to stay comfortable.

Stay away from bright lights for several hours before bedtime. Individuals might want to invest in a pair of wraparound sunglasses for the morning commute home and use dim lighting at home before going to sleep.[6]

timing for ingesting caffeine so it can enhance alertness (*see* Table 2-1 on page 27). An example of a strategic use of caffeine would be to use it after completing 8 hours of a 12-hour rotation and about 15 minutes before the start of a long surgical procedure.[8]

Although caffeine can be helpful in the short term, it does have some potential side effects of which staff members should be aware. Caffeine's side effects include the following:

Table 2-1.
The Caffeine Checklist

To help staff members use caffeine effectively, organizations should consider creating a caffeine checklist. This can help staff members determine the caffeine content of their food and drink to make sure they are ingesting healthy amounts of caffeine.

Caffeine Checklist

Tally the number of beverages consumed in a day to get your total daily caffeine consumption.

Beverage	Amount of Caffeine
8 oz. cola	23 mg
8 oz. diet cola	31 mg
240 mL Red Bull	80 mg
8 oz. coffee	110 mg
8 oz. decaf coffee	5 mg
6 oz. caffe latte	90 mg
6 oz. cappuccino	90 mg
1 oz. espresso	90 mg
1 oz. decaf espresso	10 mg
8 oz. instant coffee	90 mg
8 oz. imported tea	60 mg
8 oz. U.S. tea	60 mg
8 oz. iced tea	60 mg
1 oz. milk chocolate candy	6 mg
8 oz. cocoa beverage	6 mg

Source: Adapted from National Sleep Foundation: *The Buzz on Caffeine and Sleep*. http://www.sleepfoundation.org/atf/cf/%7BF6BF2668-A1B4-4FE8-8D1A-A5D39340D9CB%7D/caffeine.pdf (accessed Dec. 10, 2007).

- A "caffeine crash," or fatigue when the caffeine wears off
- Feelings of anxiety or irritability
- Rapid heartbeat
- Sleep disturbance due to increased time needed to fall asleep, frequent

More Information: Basic Facts About Caffeine

Caffeine is found naturally in more than 60 plants, including the coffee bean, tea leaf, kola nut, and cacao pod.[7] It is found in three popular drinks—coffee, tea, and cola—and in other soft drinks, chocolate, and some medications.

There is no nutritional need for caffeine in the diet. It enters the bloodstream through the stomach and small intestine and can have a stimulating effect as soon as 15 minutes after it is consumed. Once in the body, caffeine will persist for several hours.[7]

Caffeine is not harmful in moderation—up to 250 mg per day—as long as it is not consumed close to bedtime, which can disrupt sleep. Three 8 oz. cups of coffee per day is considered a moderate amount of caffeine. Six or more 8 oz. cups of coffee per day is considered excessive intake of caffeine.[7]

awakenings during the night, and interference in moving into the deeper, more restorative stages of sleep[9]

Individuals with high blood pressure and certain heart conditions should avoid using caffeine.

Work/Life Programs

For individuals engaging in shift work, balancing the demands of life can be quite challenging. In addition, workers who hold a second job or volunteer for overtime shifts to make ends meet can have trouble squeezing in their personal lives among all their work responsibilities. As mentioned in Chapter One, this problem can be exacerbated if the individual is also caring for young children or adult parents. To help staff members balance their work and personal responsibilities, organizations might consider increasing workers' access to work/life programs. These programs can include concierge services, such as dry-cleaning pickup, child and elder care, and access to legal or financial services, such as estate planning. Alternative work arrangements, such as job sharing and telecommuting, could also help reduce fatigue and improve morale among staff.[10]

Exercise

Like caffeine, exercise can be a stimulant, as it increases heart rate and can help an individual regain focus. Staff members who take brisk walks during their break times might be better able to combat the effects of fatigue, at least in the short term. Organizations might want to encourage such exercise, as it also provides other health and wellness benefits.

In addition to exercising during break times, staff members should be encouraged to have regular exercise routines during their personal time. Exercise options

More Information: Encouraging Good Nutrition

As mentioned in Chapter One, shift workers not only fight issues of fatigue but have an increased likelihood of suffering from obesity, cardiovascular problems, and gastrointestinal issues. This is partly due to the tendency of shift workers to eat poorly while at work. Lack of sleep can also lead to cravings for sugary and high-fat foods. Organizations can help workers address poor eating habits by providing nutritious foods in the cafeteria. Having tasty yet healthy food options—such as salads, fruits, and high-fiber carbohydrates–readily available and cost-effective can help encourage healthier eating, thus helping prevent problematic health issues.

could include walking, running, practicing yoga, and participating in sports. Organizations can help encourage exercise by supporting organizational sports teams—such as softball or basketball teams—and by providing access to a local gym.

As previously mentioned, staff members should be careful about exercising too close to the time they wish to go to sleep because exercising close to bedtime can make it more difficult to fall asleep.

Lighting and Ventilation

As previously mentioned, for individuals working the night shift, their body is fighting against the natural release of melatonin, which causes drowsiness and the urge to sleep. Light and darkness can help regulate a body's circadian rhythm and help counteract the effects of melatonin. To help workers overcome the urge to sleep, organizations should provide well-lit, well-ventilated spaces in which to work. This is an easily implemented strategy that can help improve performance as well as provider and staff safety. Some locations to consider using bright light include nurses' stations, laboratories, treatment rooms, and the emergency room. Organizations will need to consider carefully how to use light on patient floors so that it will not disturb patients who are trying to sleep.[8]

Prescription Medications

A number of safe, effective, short-acting sedative and hypnotic medications can provide improved sleep for staff members in challenging circumstances. For example, health care workers who need to sleep during the day or who have off-duty transitions between schedules might benefit from increased amount and quality of sleep, and certain prescription medications can be used to aid during these times. The use of prescription sleep medications can also reduce the amount of sleep loss experienced before a work period.[12]

Conversely, some prescription medications can help with wakefulness. Although the use of amphetamines is not allowed for clinicians because of the associated risks, one drug that has been used to aid workers with shift work is modafinil, a non-amphetamine drug that has been approved by the U.S. Food and Drug Administration (FDA) to treat narcolepsy.[13]

Staff members should consult a physician before taking any drugs to enhance wakefulness or sleepiness.

> **More Information: Cab Reimbursement**
>
> At the University of Chicago Medical Center, if an employee finishes his or her shift and feels too tired to safely drive home, there is another solution. The hospital has a cab reimbursement fund from which the hospital reimburses for cab fare home after a long shift for anyone wanting to take advantage of it. The impetus for the fund was that organization leaders were noticing anecdotally that staff members leaving the hospital after long shifts were getting into more fender benders or were commenting that they did not feel safe driving home. The hospital provides education about the program to staff members so that they know the program is available for their use any time they do not feel up to driving home.[11]

Technology

As discussed in Chapter One, when an individual is fatigued, he or she loses concentration and decision-making capability, and short-term memory is negatively affected. To counteract these detrimental affects of fatigue, organizations should consider putting in place safeguards to ensure that procedures are performed correctly despite fatigue. These safeguards might include procedural checks, such as checklists, coworker double-checks, automated reminders, and enhanced monitoring.

Computer technology can also be helpful in preventing fatigue-related errors. For example, computers can be designed to prompt for particular information and prevent incorrect information from being entered into the computer. A computerized prescriber order entry (CPOE) system can help providers enter orders clearly and accurately. It can prompt physicians to include certain information and can have fail-safe characteristics that prevent potential medication errors. Such a system helps prevent handwriting errors and can include forcing functions to prevent overdoses and potentially harmful medication interactions.

CPOE is not the only type of computer system that can help prevent fatigue-related error. Other systems, such as bar-coding systems, patient identification systems, and automated medication-dispensing systems, can help ensure that the right patient, is matched to the right medication, despite any fatigue experienced by the health care workers interacting with the patient.

Planned Naps

Although fragmented sleep is not as restorative as uninterrupted sleep, any short period of sleep, such as a brief nap, is better than none.[13] Sleep is the most effective countermeasure for sleepiness and fatigue. Consequently, brief naps can help mitigate the negative effects of sleep deprivation and fatigue, including drowsiness, impaired performance, and poor mood. Studies have shown that a 2- to 8-hour nap before 24 hours of wakefulness can improve vigilance and minimize sleepiness.[14] In addition, brief naps—lasting between 20 and 40 minutes—during a period of wakefulness can also improve performance.

Because of the clinically proven benefits of planned naps, several groups, including the Agency for Healthcare Research and Quality (AHRQ), have endorsed taking naps as a method to relieve fatigue in long work shifts.[15]

The concept of a planned nap has been tested in many industries in which workers engage in shift work or work extra-long hours. For example, field studies have shown that airline pilots and truck drivers who take a planned nap can mitigate drowsiness and improve alertness.[16] In one study conducted by the National Aeronautics and Space Administration (NASA), long-haul flight crew members who napped had significantly improved performance and alertness, including fewer microsleeps, in the last 90 minutes of flight.[17]

Some organizations might hesitate to implement a planned nap program, thinking that it might not be necessary. But data show that health care workers are fighting to stay awake on the job and are probably already napping during breaks and sometimes during the course of their work. "We know this is an issue, and we know that people are sleeping on the job," says sleep expert Mark Rosekind, Ph.D. "Isn't it better to have a planned nap than a random, uncontrolled sleep episode?"[18] A scheduled approved nap might allow workers to relax more fully and reap the full benefits of rest instead of sneaking off to take a nap with the fear of getting caught.

Overcoming Sleep Inertia

When waking from a long period of sleep, such as from a lengthy nap, individuals can experience sleep inertia. This is the fog-like state that one can experience immediately on awakening from a deep sleep. People suffering from sleep inertia may experience slowed speech, substantial performance deficits, poor memory, and impaired decision making.[14] It can take several hours to completely recover from sleep inertia, and the first 15 to 30 minutes after waking are a particularly vulnerable period. Performance during this period can be worse than that of individuals who have been awake for 24 continuous hours. Sleep inertia can be reversed with time or sufficient stimulation, such as caffeine or physical activity.[14]

Sleep inertia appears to be directly tied to the length of the sleep period. For example, sleep inertia is most likely to occur upon being woken up after a 3- to 6-hour sleep period.[14] Organizations should consider sleep inertia when designing their planned nap programs to ensure that the length of naps yields optimal performance and that the individuals waking from naps are not required to make vital decisions shortly after being woken.[19]

Making Sure Policies Support Practice

If an organization chooses to pursue a planned nap strategy, it is important to have an explicit policy that discusses this strategy. Currently, in most organizations, sleeping on the job is against the rules, and a worker can be terminated for inadvertent napping. When designing a napping policy, organizations must provide an explicit sanction of the use of planned naps in the work environment. They should also delineate specific procedures, timing, and circumstances for naps. Finally, a napping policy should address any potential concerns about misuse.[1]

Beyond policies, corporate support might include the creation of a specific nap room or space that is conducive to napping.[1] This space should be quiet, secure, and easily accessible.

Case Study 2-1.
Stanford University School of Medicine

The use of planned naps as a countermeasure to fatigue has been tested in many industries in which workers engage in shift work or work long hours. Researchers at Stanford University School of Medicine were interested in examining how planned naps could affect health care worker performance and be used as a strategy to overcome the effects of fatigue.

In June 2001, Stanford conducted a randomized, controlled intervention trial in the emergency department (ED), involving physicians and nurses. Each participant was paid, and the study was approved by the University Investigational Review Board, the ED chair, and the nurses' union.

To begin the study, Stanford recruited 49 subjects—24 nurses and 25 physicians—who worked through the night, from 7:30 P.M. to 7:30 A.M. These subjects worked in the ED of Stanford Hospital and worked at least three consecutive 12-hour night shifts. (*See* Table 2-2 on page 33)

The subjects were divided into two groups—a control group that worked straight through the night as usual and an experimental group that was allotted a 40-minute nap break at 3 A.M., in the middle of the shift. At the start of the shift,

Table 2-2.
Participant Demographics

The table shows the demographics of the participants in the study.

Characteristics	Nap Group	No-Nap Group
Mean age	30 years old	30 years old
Men	5	11
Women	21	12
Physicians	13	12
Nurses	13	11

Source: Stanford University School of Medicine, Palo Alto, California. Used with permission.

participants were not aware of which group they were in and consequently did not know whether they would be allowed a nap.

Collecting Data

Before the study began, each participant completed a background questionnaire, a sleep disorders questionnaire, a shift-work experiences questionnaire, and an Owl and Lark questionnaire (*see* Figure 2-2 on page 34). Each participant wore an electronic wrist activity monitor during the study and kept a sleep log. Participants were instructed to refrain from drinking caffeine during each night shift.

All participants scored within normal limits on the sleep disorders questionnaire and reported no evidence of clinical sleep disorders. In addition, they showed no preference for morning or evening on the Owl and Lark questionnaire.

At three points during their shift—before the shift, at the midpoint of the shift, and at the end of the shift—participants were required to take several performance tests, which took about 20 minutes. These tests included a psychomotor vigilance test—a validated 10-minute test of reaction time to evaluate simulated attention[16]—a 10-minute written memory recall test, a computer-based intravenous (IV) insertion simulation, and a questionnaire developed by NASA that measures different mood states, including anger, confusion, depression, fatigue, tension, and vigor.

At the end of their shifts, both groups also participated in a 40-minute car-drive simulation. Researchers examined videotapes of the subjects' faces while "driving." If a subject's head bobbed or his or her eyes closed for longer than 5 seconds, he or she was labeled a dangerous driver.

Figure 2-2.
Owl and Lark Questionnaire

An Owl and Lark questionnaire helps measure an individual's sleep personality—in other words, whether he or she is a "night person," a "morning person," or somewhere in between. The following are the types of questions included on an Owl and Lark questionnaire:

1. What time would you get up if you were entirely free to plan your day?
   Before 7 A.M.
   7–9 A.M.
   After 9 A.M.

2. How easy is it for you to get up on work days?
   Very difficult
   Moderately difficult/depends on the day
   Fairly easy

3. How alert do you feel during the first 30 minutes after you get up in the morning?
   Alert/fresh
   Varies
   Sleepy/tired

4. What time would you go to bed if it were completely up to you?
   After midnight
   10:30 P.M.–midnight
   Before 10:30 P.M.

5. How sleepy/tired are you 1½ hours before going to bed during the work week?
   Very tired/ready to fall asleep
   Moderately tired/depends on the day
   Not very tired

Figure 2-2. (continued)
Owl and Lark Questionnaire

6. When you've stayed up later than usual (had a late evening), when do you wake up the next morning (assuming that you didn't have any alcohol)?
   Later than usual, with a desire to fall back asleep
   Varies
   At your usual time, with a desire to get out of bed

Source: Adapted from Richard M. Coleman: *Wide Awake at 3:00 am. By Choice or by Chance.* In Horne J. A., Ostberg O.: A self assesment questionnaire to determine morningness-eveningness in human circadian rhythms. *International Journal of Chronobiology* 4:97–110, 1976.

The Nap

For those individuals who were allowed to nap, the nap took place in a dark, quiet room away from clinical sites. A bed with linens was provided. Each individual was allowed a 40-minute nap opportunity. During the nap, participants were wired with electroencephalogram (EEG) and electriculography (EOG) monitors to check the quality of the nap.

Results of the Study

Before the planned nap, both the control group and experimental group showed degrading performance as their shifts progressed. However, after the nap, the performance of the experimental group remained constant, whereas the control group's performance continued to decline. Consequently, the group that napped scored fewer performance lapses and reported more vigor, less fatigue, and less sleepiness. The physicians and nurses who napped also tended to complete the simulated IV insertion more quickly and showed fewer behavioral signs of sleepiness while driving.

Interestingly, the nap did not seem to have an effect on the individuals' driving ability after the shift. Both the control and experimental groups had a substantial number of lapses in driving during the simulation, such as leaving the road or colliding with an oncoming vehicle. The researchers hypothesized that the nap occurred too early in the shift to effect postshift driving performance, and if a nap is taken postshift before driving, improved safety in driving might be realized.

"One of the interesting things about this study is that many of the participants indicated that they didn't think they could fall asleep at work, and yet 90% of participants in the experimental group napped, and the average nap time was approximately

25 minutes," says Rebecca Smith-Coggins, M.D., associate professor of surgery/emergency medicine for Stanford. "Those individuals in the experimental group fell asleep very quickly, some in less than 10 minutes."

After their nap, the group scored lower on a probed memory recall task than the group that stayed awake. This might have been due to sleep inertia, which usually clears in 5 to 10 minutes.

The Stanford nap study was the first randomized trial of a nap intervention during the night shift for physicians and nurses. The study ultimately showed that a 40-minute nap opportunity allows health care professionals to maintain their performance, alertness, and mood through the end of their shift.

Case Study 2-2.
VA Palo Alto Health Care System

The Veterans Administration (VA) has long been at the forefront of addressing patient safety issues, including worker fatigue. The VA's National Center for Patient Safety (NCPS) is working on a planned nap program, to be implemented across all 170 VA facilities in the United States.

The idea of a planned nap program was started at the VA facility in Palo Alto, California, near the campus of Stanford University. Steven K. Howard, M.D., director of the Patient Safety Center of Inquiry for VA Palo Alto Health Care System, had been involved in the Stanford University nap study (*see* Case Study 2-1 on page 32) and wanted to see how a planned nap program could improve performance at his organization.

Before implementing the program, Howard talked with organization leadership, including the chief medical officer and the director of the hospital, as well as other stakeholders in the project, such as physicians and nurses working on the units, representatives from the union, and human resources representatives. He received support and buy-in from all participants and went forward with the project. "Organization leaders acknowledged that fatigue was a problem in our hospital and were supportive of efforts to try to reduce worker fatigue and improve patient and provider safety," says Howard.

The organization began the program by implementing it within the medical/surgical intensive care unit (ICU) and the intermediate ICU of the hospital. Howard chose the two ICU units to pilot test the program because they are of high medical acuity, errors are known to occur in these settings, and workers in these areas had high intrinsic interest in the project. The organization particularly wanted to focus on the nursing staff with this initiative. "Taking a quick nap while on call is not unusual for physicians, but up until this point, it had been unheard of for nurses. It required a big shift in thinking for all members of the organization," says Howard.

As a first step in the program, VA Palo Alto offered education and information to the physicians and nurses on the units about sleep deprivation and fatigue. The Microsoft PowerPoint educational component was 15 to 20 minutes long, introduced the concept of fatigue, and suggested napping as a strategy to combat fatigue. At the end of the training, participants signed an agreement showing that they were willing to try the napping exercise and would not abuse it.

Each participant was also provided with a personal use tool, which described how to plan and execute a strategic nap (*see* Figure 2-3, below). This tool describes the four P's of an effective nap experience (*See* Appendix Three for another tool example.):

- Planning
- Prenap preparation
- Place
- Postnap recovery

Figure 2-3.
The VA Strategic Nap Program: Personal Use Tool

As part of the strategic nap program, VA Palo Alto provided physicians and nurses in the two intensive care units with a personal use tool, the content of which is shown here. This tool takes the form of a 3" x 5" spiral-bound booklet that workers can carry in their pockets.

Need a Nap?
How would you know? Consider the following questions to help you decide:

- How long was your last sleep period?
- How long have you been awake?
- Are you working in the middle of the night?
- Is your schedule regular?
- Do you feel tired or sleepy?
- Have you noticed any problems with your memory or attention?
- Have you noticed any changes in your actions (for example, slowed reaction time)?
- Have you been nodding off?

(continued)

Figure 2-3. (continued)
The VA Strategic Nap Program: Personal Use Tool

If your answers to the questions above suggest that you are tired or sleepy, then a strategic nap may benefit you. Follow the four P's provided here to help you use a strategic nap: plan, prenap, place, and postnap.

Plan

Have a plan for your nap.

How long?

- For a short nap: ≤ 45 minutes
  For a longer nap: ≤ 2 hours
- Be sure not to take a long nap too close to your next planned sleep period.
- Getting some sleep is better than no sleep.

When?

- Be clear on beginning and end times—don't leave it open-ended.

Wake-up plan?

- Establish a specific and reliable mechanism for awakening (for example, an alarm clock or a specific person to wake you).

Prenap

Team communication and coordination

Handoff prenap

- Inform others of nap plan.
- Hand off appropriate clinical information.

Emergency callback

- Identify mechanism for callback.
- Identify potential clinical situations that may require attention.

Place

Environmental/facility checklist

- Use a dark, quiet, cool room and a comfortable sleep surface.
- Consider using an eye shade or earplugs.
- Consider using white noise.
- Address privacy/security issues.
- Use a wake-up mechanism that is reliable and easy to use.

Figure 2-3. (continued)
The VA Strategic Nap Program: Personal Use Tool

Postnap

Wake up

- Allow yourself a wake-up period.
- You may want to stretch, move around, generally be physically active, turn on the lights, and increase social interaction.

Handoff postnap

- Get back into "the loop" with an update regarding clinical status.
- Increase team interaction and monitoring while becoming fully integrated back into clinical activities.

Source: VA Palo Alto Health System, Palo Alto, California. Used with permission.

Since the planned nap program was implemented, the organization has also provided access to online resources to answer any questions physicians and nurses might have about the physiology of sleep and the research associated with fatigue and planned napping. The organization also provides staff with access to some examples of when a strategic nap would be appropriate (*see* "More Information: When to Use a Planned Nap" on page 40).

Before implementing the planned nap program, VA Palo Alto created a designated spot for napping. This is a quiet, secure place that is close to the two ICUs. It is about a 90-second walk from where care is provided. The room has a bed with linens and a bathroom. "One issue we have with this room is that the perception is it is too far away from the clinical areas. Staff members are sometimes still taking their naps in the break room instead of walking the extra distance to the nap room," says Howard. The organization is working to educate staff on the benefits of using the napping room in order to further encourage use.

To measure the success of the nap program implementation, Howard engaged in walk-arounds, where he asked staff members how the naps were going. He identified whether the staff members were taking naps and, if not, why. He also had participants fill out sleep logs, and he examined those logs to determine whether people were napping.

The results of VA Palo Alto's program have been positive. Staff members are pleased with the nap concept and take advantage of it. They also communicate with organization leadership their appreciation for the program. "When you have a

More Information: When to Use a Planned Nap

The following examples are provided by the National Center for Patient Safety, Ann Arbor, Michigan, as good times to take planned naps.

Jim works the night shift and is scheduled for a 12-hour shift tonight, beginning at 1900 hours. He missed his usual opportunity to sleep in the afternoon at home because his infant child was sick and crying. His usual practice was to obtain 2 to 3 hours of sleep before coming in to work. His shift tonight will be his third in a row, but he feels pretty good. Around midnight of his shift, he is feeling tired and asks his supervisor if he can take his 30-minute break a little early. The unit is busy, but his supervisor assesses the situation and decides to let Jim go. After giving a report on his patients, Jim lets his supervisor know that he is going to use his break for a nap and says he will set his alarm in order to wake up. Jim estimates that he got about 25 minutes of sleep during his break. He integrates back into the unit after getting a verbal report from the covering nurse.

Ana is an intern working in the intensive care unit. She is paired with Sara, who is an internal medicine resident, and they are on call every third night. The unit has been particularly busy this month, and Ana thinks she will easily push 80 hours per week for the 4-week rotation. She and Sara are on call, and they planned their night to each take a 45-minute nap during the course of their call to maintain alertness. During the nap, the covering physician will carry the other's pager so they will not be bothered. Each will be responsible for waking the other one. Before each nap, they brief each other on what tasks need to be performed while the other one sleeps. Sara is the first to nap, at 0100, and she estimates that she slept for 40 minutes. Ana goes for her nap at 0230. Sara let Ana sleep for 2 hours.

Jeff and Beth are the surgical house staff on call. Jeff is an intern who is covering all calls, allowing Beth to take a nap. They planned to each get a 2-hour nap over the course of their call. About an hour after Beth goes to her call room, the code pager goes off. Jeff wakes Beth, and they run to the code together.

Melissa, a recent graduate from nursing school, has worked the night shift for the past 6 months. She is not particularly fond of the night shift but is trying her best to adapt. She notes that after each consecutive night shift, she feels progressively more fatigued. At 0700 on Friday (the end of her fourth consecutive night shift), she is very sleepy. She decides to take a short nap before her 30-minute commute home.

frontline staff person expressing enthusiasm and telling organization leaders how much he or she benefits from a nap, it can go a long way toward maintaining leadership buy-in," says Howard.

A nap program has been successfully implemented at the VA facility in Portland, Oregon. "When designing a nap program, organizations need to look at their own staff needs, resources, and culture. The program at VA Portland is different from the [VA Palo Alto] program, but both programs work in the particular environments in which they were started," says Howard. The NCPS is hard at work helping the other VA sites around the country implement customized nap programs. "It may be a long process, but we are hopeful that one day soon every VA site will have a planned nap program that works in its organization," says Howard.

Case Study 2-3.
University of Chicago Hospitals

For many interns who work 30-hour shifts, the use of a planned nap could be of great benefit. In 2003, University of Chicago Hospitals (UCH) began a study to see if intern performance would increase as a result of a planned nap and to determine whether instituting a planned nap during a 30-hour shift could provide another option for limiting the schedule for physicians-in-training.

Within the confines of the study, for two weeks of their general medicine rotations, a selected number of interns could take naps while on duty. For the other two weeks, these interns had standard schedules. A resident physician on night-float service provided coverage between midnight and 7:00 A.M. so interns could finish their work and take naps. Although coverage was not mandatory, interns on the nap schedule were strongly encouraged to forward the care of their patients to the night-float physician.

To collect data, UCH used activity monitors worn around each intern's wrist, which detected the participants' movement. From these monitors, researchers were able to study sleep efficiency and quality. They looked at the interns' self-reported levels of fatigue and reviewed paging logs to determine how often interns forwarded their pagers to the night-float resident. An investigator privately interviewed all interns, without previous notification of the purpose of the interview. The investigator asked interns whether they preferred the nap schedule or the regular schedule when they were on call and why. In addition, the investigator asked the interns which schedule they preferred for their patients when they were not on call.

The Results

The UHC nap schedule resulted in modest increases in sleep for the participating interns over the standard schedule. In addition, interns on the nap schedule reported significant reduction in fatigue on the postcall day. The study showed that call-night coverage that allows even modest increases in sleep can reduce fatigue.

Interns with a nap schedule slept for about 3 hours. Interns with the nap schedule who forwarded their pagers to the night-float physician could receive protected sleep time. The amount of protected sleep time was significantly associated with on-call sleep. For each hour that an intern was covered, the intern received 42 minutes of additional sleep. For example, interns who forwarded their pagers to the night-float physician slept for an average of 5.7 hours, whereas those who did not forward their pagers slept for 3.9 hours. The gap probably occurred because interns stayed awake to finish work.

Most interns cited that they preferred the nap schedule when they were on call because the schedule improved sleep, decreased fatigue, and provided a greater ability to focus on care for their own patients because of the reduced workload of cross-coverage. Ironically, the overwhelming majority of these same interns wished that their patients were not cared for on the nap schedule during periods when they were not on call.

One interesting point revealed in this study was that interns have an intense desire to continue to care for their own patients and often opted to take shorter naps to do so. Interns on the nap schedule forwarded their pagers to the night-float physician on only 22% of available opportunities. In lieu of forwarding their pagers, interns with the nap schedule preferred to forward the care of only their crossover patients and to retain care of their own patients.

In addition, interns expressed concern about handoff communications and continuity of care within the napping program. "When designing a planned nap program, organizations will need to address continuity of care issues and make sure physicians feel comfortable transferring their patients into someone else's care," says Vineet Arora, M.D., associate program director for the internal medicine residency at UCH.

UCH is in the process of implementing the planned nap option across its facility. It is also working on implementing cultural changes that will support the nap program, such as education on fatigue and sleep deprivation, a cab reimbursement program, and a standardized handoff communication initiative.

Diagnosing and Treating Sleep Disorders

Nearly 40 million American men and women suffer from sleep disorders, and there are almost 90 different disorders that can be diagnosed and treated.[1] Undiagnosed sleep disorders can be a significant issue for health care organizations, as they can cause excessive fatigue and performance issues among affected workers and can introduce risks to patient and provider safety. For this reason, any alertness management program should also include a method of acquainting staff with the different sleep disorders and of encouraging staff to seek professional advice if they have concerns about a particular sleep disorder.

Staff members should be trained on different sleep disorders and how to recognize the signs of common disorders. Organizations should consider providing information about accredited sleep disorder clinics available for referral and possibly extending insurance coverage for these services.[1] If a staff person shows the symptoms of a sleep disorder, he or she should be empowered to seek the opinion of a medical professional.

The following sections briefly describe some of the most common sleep disorders.

Insomnia

Insomnia is the most common sleep problem.[20] It is a condition in which individuals have trouble falling asleep or staying asleep. Some people with insomnia fall asleep easily but wake up before they want to. Other people have the opposite problem, or they have trouble both falling asleep and staying asleep. The end result is poor-quality sleep that doesn't leave an individual feeling refreshed when he or she wakes up.[21]

More than half of the American public (63% of women and 54% of men) experience symptoms of insomnia at least a few nights a week.[20] There are two main types of insomnia: The most common type is called *secondary insomnia*, and more than 8 out of 10 people with insomnia have this type.[21] *Secondary insomnia* is a symptom or a side effect of some other problem. Some of the problems that can cause secondary insomnia include the following:

- Certain illnesses, such as some heart and lung diseases
- Pain, anxiety, and depression
- Medicines that delay or disrupt sleep as a side effect
- Caffeine, tobacco, alcohol, and other substances that affect sleep
- Another sleep disorder, such as restless legs syndrome (RLS)
- A poor sleep environment
- A change in sleep routine

In contrast, primary insomnia is not a side effect of medicines or another medical problem. It is its own disorder and generally persists for at least a month.[21]

Insomnia can cause excessive daytime sleepiness and a lack of energy. Long-term insomnia can cause depression and irritability and can result in difficulties paying attention, learning, and remembering.[21]

Fortunately, healthy sleep habits—such as regular bedtimes and waking times, exercise, and dietary changes—can help improve insomnia. If an individual's insomnia persists, and lifestyle, behavioral, or diet changes do not help, a physician might prescribe a sleep-promoting medication. If there is an underlying and treat-

More Information: Why Do People Snore?

Snoring is defined as "breathing during sleep with hoarse or harsh sounds as caused by the vibrating of the soft palate." Although people often joke about whether they snore and how loudly they snore, snoring is no laughing matter. It can be a marker of sleep apnea or a risk factor for vascular complications, such as hypertension. It can lead to daytime dysfunction due to the fragmented sleep that can result from snoring.

Snoring can cause headaches, difficulty with concentration, fatigue, and reduced work performance. Snoring can also annoy family members, whose sleep quality can be affected by their loved one's snoring.[20]

There are many different ways to reduce snoring and one of the most effective is through weight loss in overweight individuals. By reducing weight, an individual will reduce fat deposits in the throat, providing a more spacious airway and usually less snoring. Another way to reduce snoring is to improve nasal breathing by using a nasal strip that gently opens the nostrils during sleep. Dental appliances are also available that can help reduce snoring. Sleeping on the side with a pillow is the preferable position to help alleviate snoring.[20]

Two further lifestyle changes to consider to reduce snoring are avoiding alcohol and cigarettes. Abstaining from alcohol, which relaxes the muscles in the airway, at least four hours before bedtime and abstaining completely from smoking, which is associated with nasal congestion, can help alleviate snoring.[20]

able cause of the insomnia, such as depression, stress, anxiety, reflux, bladder problems, or pain, a physician might prescribe antidepressants; anxiolytics (anti-anxiety drugs); medications for heartburn, incontinence, or pain; and/or hypnotic medications to improve sleep.[20]

Sleep Apnea

Sleep apnea is a serious sleep disorder in which an individual's breathing periodically stops or becomes shallow during sleep. These pauses in breathing can last for 10 to 20 seconds and can occur 20 to 30 times per hour. With the most common type of sleep apnea, obstructive sleep apnea, not enough air flows into the lungs during sleep. When this happens, the amount of oxygen in the blood can drop. The brain emits adrenaline to wake up the body and resume normal breathing. This is characterized by a loud snort or choking sound. When the breathing pauses occur, the body moves out of deep sleep into light sleep, resulting in poor sleep quality. This, in turn, can result in excessive daytime sleepiness.[22]

An estimated 18 million Americans have sleep apnea. Studies have found that untreated sleep apnea is associated with increased blood pressure, a risk for cardiovascular disease, and stroke.[20] Untreated sleep apnea can also increase the risk of diabetes and the risk for work-related accidents and driving accidents.[22] People with untreated sleep apnea are six times more likely to have a car crash than individuals without sleep apnea.[18]

People with sleep apnea often have loud snoring. However, not everyone who snores has sleep apnea. Sleep apnea happens more often in people who are overweight, but thin people can experience it as well. Most people don't know they have sleep apnea. A family member and/or bed partner might notice the signs of sleep apnea first.[22]

The good news about sleep apnea is that it can be treated. Sleeping masks and surgery are just some of the options available to address the problem. When sleep apnea is treated, the risks of adverse health effects and driving accidents return to normal levels.

RLS and Periodic Limb Movement Disorder (PLMD)

RLS is a neurological movement disorder affecting as many as 12 million Americans.[20] It is a sensory disorder that causes an almost irresistible urge to move the legs. The urge to move is usually due to unpleasant feelings in the legs that occur when at rest. People with RLS use words such as *creeping*, *crawling*, *tingling*, and *burning* to describe these feelings. Moving the legs eases the feelings, but only for a while.[23]

People who suffer from RLS can have difficulty sleeping, daytime sleepiness, mood swings, anxiety, and depression. One study found that 42% of those with RLS stated that it affected their relationship with their partner.[20] RLS can range from mild to severe, based on the following factors:

- The amount of leg discomfort
- The need to move around
- The amount of relief received from moving around
- The amount of sleep disturbance
- The resulting sleepiness
- Frequency of symptoms
- Severity of symptoms
- The impact on daily life
- The effect on the individual's mood and personality

Although the exact cause of RLS is not known, recent research indicates that iron or folate deficiency might be a risk factor. Treatments include iron or vitamin supplements, lifestyle changes, and medications.[20]

About 80% of those with RLS also have PLMD, or involuntary leg twitching or jerking movements during sleep that can occur every 20 to 30 seconds.[20] These movements cause repeated awakenings that disturb or reduce sleep. PLMD usually affects the legs but can also affect the arms.[23]

Narcolepsy

Narcolepsy is a chronic neurological disorder that affects approximately 1 in 2,000 people.[20] It causes a person to have difficulty staying awake and can cause a person to suddenly fall asleep during the day. These "sleep attacks" occur even after getting enough sleep at night and can involve a loss in muscle tone or strength. The unusual sleep pattern that people with narcolepsy have can affect their schooling, work, and social life.[24]

People with narcolepsy often fall asleep without warning at inappropriate times. Sleep attacks don't just happen during quiet times, such as when reading or watching TV. These attacks can occur during driving, eating, or other activities and can cause accidents and injuries, as well as impaired memory, thinking, or ability to concentrate.[24] Recent scientific breakthroughs have led to new understanding of the cause of this condition, and new treatments have given physicians more ways to help manage its symptoms.[20]

Scheduling to Reduce Fatigue

Changing work schedules, including limiting work hours, is how many industries besides health care that battle with fatigue issues are addressing the problem. The most widely used approach across industries that need to address worker fatigue is to regulate "hours of service" (HOS).[1] These regulations typically establish specific requirements intended to provide rest opportunities and duty time limitations to prevent extended periods of work and wakefulness. Such an approach might also address total work hours in a certain number of days or an identified number of days off for recovery. In addition, such regulations might establish a specific work time within a duty period; for example, in trucking, commercial drivers can only have a certain drive time during a particular duty period. In aviation, a pilot may have a specific flight time associated with a duty period.[1]

Scheduling is probably the most difficult and potentially contentious component of an alertness management program. Individuals who have worked for a health care organization for a long time may be used to the schedule and unwilling to change. They might feel that newer members of the organization are "getting off easy" and, without the proper education on the need for healthy sleep and impact of fatigue, might not support schedule changes. For this reason, it is critical to implement scheduling changes with other solutions, such as education and alertness strategies. If everyone in the organization is aware of and understands the problem and effects of sleep deprivation and fatigue, there is greater likelihood that schedule changes will be supported.

When considering changes to a work schedule, health care organizations should keep in mind that fatigue is affected by the number of hours an individual works, the particular shift he or she works, the number of work days scheduled before a day off, and the number of days off before returning to work (*see* Sidebar 2-1, below).[25]

Several scheduling options are available to health care organizations, including fixed schedules or rotating shifts. Fixed schedules are permanent, and staff members volunteer to work the same schedule—day, evening, or night—on a permanent basis. Although these types of shifts allow a worker's circadian rhythm to adjust and can lead to better performance, daytime commitments and social obligations often prevent workers from completely adapting to permanent night shifts, and this can affect worker satisfaction.[26]

Rotating schedules can rotate quickly or slowly, forward or backward.[12] Ideally, schedules should rotate forward to follow the circadian rhythm. In other words, shifts should move from morning to evening to night, as opposed to the other way around. Forward rotation is easier to tolerate physiologically because the natural circadian rhythm tends to move forward, and it is more difficult to fall asleep earlier than the normal bedtime.[25]

When designing rotating schedules, an organization should also consider the speed of the rotation. A slow rotation—changing from one shift to another every one to two weeks—might allow better adaptation of the circadian rhythm than fast rotation—changing shifts every two to three days.

Changing work schedules can also include limiting work hours. For example, organizations might want to change schedules to accommodate 8-hour shifts instead of 12-hour shifts to reduce the likelihood of fatigue-related errors. Organizations might opt to limit work hours and increase the number of days

Sidebar 2-1. Factors to Consider in Designing Work Schedules

- Shift length
- Work time within duty period
- Consecutive workdays
- Recovery opportunities
- Work cycles of days on and days off
- Start and end times of duty periods
- Day-to-night duty transitions
- Overtime of extended-duty periods
- On-call or reserve status and procedures
- Duty and recovery opportunities over extended periods[12]

per week an individual works in order to give the individual more time off between shifts. To be effective, organizations must have well-rested staff members available to relieve those ending shifts. Organizations might need to add more staff to accommodate reductions in work hours.

Because 8 hours is the recommended amount of sleep for most adults, organizations must recognize the importance of scheduling 12 hours off work between shifts. This allows individuals to address any personal needs before getting a healthy amount of sleep. Likewise, a 24-hour time period is recommended between shifts for those who rotate shifts.[25]

In addition to scheduling shorter hours and appropriate shifts, organizations should make sure that staff meetings are not scheduled in the morning for those individuals working the night shift.[25] They should also limit the use of mandatory overtime to emergencies. No one can foresee when a natural or other disaster will necessitate staff members being present, but the cumulative effects of consecutive shifts, regular overtime, and unscheduled overtime can seriously weaken staff members' ability to perform their duties correctly and safely.

Whatever method of scheduling an organization chooses to pursue, it is important to involve staff in designing the schedule. Ideally, within each unit or area, workers should have some degree of flexibility in choosing shifts.[8]

Technologies are available that can help develop optimal schedules to reduce fatigue. One such tool, called the Fatigue Avoidance Scheduling Tool (FAST), is currently being tested by the Federal Railroad Administration (*see* Sidebar 2-2 on page 49)

Addressing the Performance of Certain Tasks

When developing a schedule for health care workers, organizations might not have much choice. There are certain times when extended shifts are either unavoidable or necessary. To address fatigue-associated risks during these times, organizations should identify tasks that might no longer be performed by individuals after extended duty hours or by individuals who are assessed to be at a performance-degrading level of fatigue. These tasks might include those that require swift and accurate action, such as ED care or rapid response team intervention, or those that require complex thinking, such as mathematical calculations or diagnostic analyses. A review of commonly performed tasks can help identify those that should be limited. In certain cases, tests can be performed to determine whether workers are too fatigued to continue caring for patients. This should not be a punitive system, in which fatigued workers are fearful of reprisal. Rather, the focus should be on completing tasks correctly for the sake of patient safety and high-quality care.

Sidebar 2-2. Fatigue Avoidance Scheduling Tool (FAST)

Developed by a human performance research firm, FAST is based on the Sleep, Activity, Fatigue, and Task Effectiveness (SAFTE) model, developed by the Department of Defense. SAFTE uses current research on how time of day and sleep/wake patterns influence cognitive capacity and risk of performance error. FAST works in the following two ways:

1. Users can enter potential work schedules prospectively to determine whether they will provide a worker with adequate rest.

2. Users can enter an actual work/sleep schedule retrospectively, following an adverse event, to determine whether fatigue was a likely factor.

FAST was originally developed for the U.S. Air Force and U.S. Army, and it is currently being tested by the Federal Railroad Administration. "We just finished a validation and calibration study of FAST, and we have a high level of confidence in the accuracy of this tool," says Ralph L. Elston, director, human performance programs for the Federal Railroad Administration in Fort Worth, Texas. "We've been encouraging railroads to use scientific methodologies in scheduling, and this seems to be a good solution. I've run more than 100 simulations with it, and I've learned a lot about how to develop schedules that work with people's circadian rhythms." Elston notes that whereas it is primarily being used in the areas of defense and transportation, FAST could have applications in other high-risk work environments, such as health care.

More Information: The Effects of Moonlighting

One major hurdle involved with scheduling is moonlighting. A lot of people who work in health care also work second jobs. The nursing shortage means there is a lot of extra work available, and, as previously mentioned, people who have financial concerns see moonlighting as an opportunity to earn more money. So, an organization might limit the hours scheduled for a particular individual, but if that person leaves the organization and works another eight-hour shift somewhere else, he or she will be fatigued.

Unfortunately, organizations can do little to address this problem other than to educate staff on the hazards of working extra shifts and provide increased compensation, benefits, and incentives to discourage the practice of moonlighting.

More Information: Scheduling Resident Duty Hours

As discussed in Chapter One, the Accreditation Council for Graduate Medical Education (ACGME) has established standards on the number of duty hours residents can work, which amount to no more than 80 hours per week averaged across 4 weeks. There are many different approaches to addressing the ACGME requirements. Researchers at McGaw Medical Center at Northwestern University developed the following four methods, which allow residents to not exceed the duty hour requirements while still maintaining an exemplary level of education.[27]

The Stretch Model. This type of scheduling requires residents to be on call every fourth night and to leave early the morning after their call shifts have ended. Although this limits the workweek and allows opportunities for reading, it has no other significant educational advantages.

The Night-Float Model. This model involves a traditional resident team and designates a certain percentage of the team to work the night shift for a period of time, such as a month. The night shift overlaps with the day shift by a significant time period in order to ensure effective communication and patient handoff.

The Apprentice Model. This model pairs a resident with one or two faculty members with whom he or she works exclusively. When the faculty member(s) is on call, the resident is also on call. This model allows for maximum educational benefit and also maintains an appropriate amount of duty hours.

The Case-Based Model. This model involves assigning residents to patient cases based on each resident's learning needs. Residents meet once a week to receive assignments and determine which attending they will be working with during the particular week, based on the case assignments. Proficiency with patient care is assessed through a formal assessment process.

Avoiding Communication Errors

One of the challenges associated with adjusting work schedules is the balance between well-rested workers and workers who are informed about the patients. For example, physicians working shorter continuous periods of clinical duty might be more rested, have better judgment, and make better clinical decisions; however, the physicians working longer shifts might have greater knowledge and understanding of the patients they have been observing for many hours and thus might make better clinical decisions.[28]

Although limiting work hours, changing work schedules, and implementing a nap program can significantly reduce issues associated with sleep deprivation and fatigue, these measures can introduce a new problem that can be just as problematic and can have just as great an impact on patient safety. Because all these strategies require more individuals to have contact with a patient, a communication issue between care providers can arise. In other words, the same physician or nurse is no longer following a patient throughout his or her care, but his or her care is being managed by multiple providers on different shifts. Without proper communication procedures, transitions between clinicians can be problematic, but if the transitions are managed properly, continuity of care can be ensured.[13]

The good news is that the problems associated with multiple providers can be easily addressed if organizations put systems in place to address them. An important system to implement is one that addresses handoff communications. To improve care, organizations should standardize handoff communications and include an opportunity to ask and respond to questions. More information about improving communication to prevent fatigue-related errors can be found in Chapter Three.

Case Study 2-4.
Jackson Memorial Hospital

With 225,000 emergency and urgent care visits and 60,000 admissions per year, Jackson Memorial Hospital, located in Miami, Florida, is a busy place. Several years ago, the process of admitting patients from the ED to inpatient beds was at its breaking point. The increasing number of admissions combined with new regulations from the ACGME and the Residency Review Committee (RRC)—which limit the number of hours a resident or an intern can work during a particular call and limit the number of patients that a resident can treat while on call—yielded an environment where there were more people needing to be admitted than the current staff was allowed to handle on a particular day.

"Because of the regulations, a fixed number of admissions were being admitted to a fixed number of services within a shorter period of the day. As a result, many patients were being held in the ED for as long as 15 hours before internal medicine saw the patient or wrote admission orders," says Aman Sabharwal, M.D., formerly one of two nocturnists for Jackson Memorial Hospital, now the associate medical director for Inpatient Services. "Patients would be held overnight in the ED until they could be admitted the next morning. This created not only an unpleasant situation for patients but a safety issue as well."

Comfort and safety weren't the only concerns. "One of our other concerns was that ED physicians were caring for patients who were essentially inpatients while continuing to treat new ED patients," says Sabharwal. "ED physicians aren't specifically trained in internal medicine, and yet these physicians were caring for patients who required that type of care. This became a quality-of-care issue as well as a safety issue for the hospital."

In an attempt to address these safety and quality-of-care issues, Jackson Memorial Hospital created the Emergency Medical Hospitalist Service (EMHS), otherwise known as a nocturnist service. The goals of this service are to provide attending-level care to patients requiring admission, allow the hospital to operate within the admission cap guidelines set forth by the RRC, and allow the admissions process to continue during the time in which the ACGME work-hour limits affect the hospital.

How the Nocturnist Service Works

The nocturnist service at Jackson Memorial Hospital is staffed by two physicians trained in internal medicine. Each evening at 8 P.M., one of the two nocturnists arrives at the hospital and admits any ED patients who are waiting to be admitted to the hospital. The nocturnist performs the necessary history and physical, writes admission orders, identifies an open bed for the patient, and begins treatment. The nocturnist uses a special admission order sheet that helps streamline the admissions process (*see* Figure 2-4 on page 53).

To help quickly identify a bed for the patient, the nocturnist communicates, sometimes via two-way radio, with one of the organization's patient placement coordinators. The patient placement coordinator position, now in its fifth year of implementation, facilitates prompt bed assignment and movement of patients to in-house beds. The position is filled by senior nurses with strong administrative and clinical backgrounds whose sole job is to improve ED throughput, improve bed utilization throughout the hospital, and ensure that patients are assigned to in-house settings that will provide the appropriate level of care.

In addition to admitting patients at the start of the shift, the nocturnist admits any new patients who require admission to the hospital throughout the night. "As soon as the ED physician makes the decision to admit a patient, the nocturnist interviews and examines the patient and writes admission orders," says Sabharwal. "This speeds up the process of the patient's evaluation and allows the patient to be immediately transferred to an assigned in-house bed." During a typical 12-hour shift, the nocturnist admits 10 to 12 new patients. "Admitting patients in the evening assures a better night's rest for the patients and improves the hospital's bed utilization," say Sabharwal. "The nocturnist treats the patients throughout the night, ordering tests and addressing any needs they may have."

Just before the end of the shift, usually between 6 A.M. and 8 A.M., the nocturnist signs out his or her patients to the appropriate medical professional. Depending on the patient, this could be the daytime hospitalist, a resident, or a specialty service. In some cases, a patient can be discharged at the end of the shift. Before signing

Figure 2-4.
Nocturnist Special Admission Order Form

DATE/TIME	***Circle desired orders.*** ***Only circled orders will be carried out.***	HUS INIT	TECH INIT	RN INIT	TIME
	Note: *Inpatient systemic antimicrobial medications must be ordered on a "Physician's Antimicrobial Order Form for Inpatients"*				
	1. Admit to Emergency Medical Hospitalist Service. Pager ________ Dr. ____________________ @ ____________ Dr. ____________________ @ ____________				
	2. Admit to ER-H / Reg. Med Surg Bed / Tele / Isolation				
	3. At 7:00, Transfer to Medical Team ____________ Attending: ________________ Resident: ________________ Intern: ________________ Pager: ________________				
	4. Diagnosis:				
	5. Allergies:				
	6. Condition:				
	7. Vital signs every _____ hours				
	8. Finger stick glucose every _____ hours				
	9. Call physician if: heart rate below 50 or above 100; respiratory rate above 24; temperature above 100.9; systolic blood pressure below 90 or above 160; oxygen saturation below 90				
	10. Activity: bed rest or bed rest with bathroom privileges as tolerated or turn every ____ hours				
	11. Strict intake and output; cardiac monitor; pulse oximetry				
	12. Precautions: delirium tremens; seizure; aspiration				
	13. Diet: nothing by mouth; regular; clear liquid; low sodium; American Diabetic Association; other ______________________________				
	14. IV: Heplock (0.9 sodium chloride or dextrose 5% and 0.45 sodium chloride) or bolus __________ mL over ________ or ________________				
	15. Medications:				
	A. E.				
	B. F.				
	C. G.				
	D. H.				
	16. Oxygen _____ L per minute via nasal cannula or _________ respiratory treatments: (see Respiratory Therapy Order Form)				
	17. Stat labs:				
	18. Obtain cardiac enzymes and ECG every 6 hours for a total of 3 sets				
	19. Imaging studies:				
	20. Morning labs:				
	______________________________ Physician's Signature and ID #				

Signature/Title	Initials	Signature/Title	Initials	Signature/Title	Initials

PHARMACY ORDERS MUST CONTAIN
NAME OF MEDICATION — DOSE — STRENGTH
ROUTE — FREQUENCY
JACKSON HEALTH SYSTEM
MIAMI, FLORIDA 33136

PATIENT IMPRINT

C-290HG	**EMERGENCY MEDICINE HOSPITALIST SERVICE PHYSICIAN ORDERS**

REV 2/04

Source: Jackson Memorial Hospital, Miami, Florida. Used with permission.

out a patient, the nocturnist also checks on any ordered laboratory studies and other diagnostic tests.

Gaining Support for the Program

Initially, the Jackson Memorial ED staff put up some resistance to the program. "As with any other new initiative, there was some pushback; however, once ED staff members saw the benefits to their patients—safer, higher-quality, and more efficient care—they began to embrace the program," says Sabharwal.

The program was sold to hospital administration by pointing out the patient safety and revenue benefits. "The hospital cannot bill for holding patients in the ED. If we admit patients and move them to an inpatient bed, the hospital can generate otherwise lost revenue," says Sabharwal. "Our billings and collections have shown that the nocturnist program not only pays for itself but also generates additional funds for the hospital." The program has worked so well that the hospital has implemented a daytime hospitalist service to help with admissions and patient care during the day.

Benefits of the Nocturnist Program

On a system level, the nocturnist program at Jackson Memorial Hospital has improved ED throughput and inpatient bed use. "The program also allows the hospital to comply with the ACGME and RRC regulations without negatively impacting patients," says Sabharwal. "Patients are not forced to sit and wait to be admitted but can begin their treatment right away. Patients receive the most appropriate treatment in a timely manner, which can improve their quality of care, decrease their length of stay, and improve their satisfaction." Because the nocturnist is in the hospital when admitting patients, the program allows for a more precise and accurate history and physical, diagnosis, and treatment plan. "Physicians who are on call at home often do not get the complete or correct story from the ED, which can sometimes lead to incomplete admission orders, unnecessary tests, and delayed treatment plans," says Sabharwal. "Because the nocturnist actually examines the patient, there is less likelihood for error."

In addition to the benefits to the patient, the nocturnist program at Jackson Memorial also benefits the staff. The nocturnists themselves, because they work only at night and are not alternating between the day and night shifts, experience less fatigue and stress. Due to their consistent waking and sleeping schedule, they are more alert and less likely to make mistakes. The two nocturnists have designed their own schedule, following a one-week-on, one-week-off routine. The burden is also lifted from ED staff members, who can focus more of their attention on ED patients requiring their services.

Although a hospital cannot control the number of patients who walk through the door needing admission, it can control the process of admission. By implementing a nocturnist service, Jackson Memorial Hospital has streamlined the admission process and enhanced patient safety and quality of care at the same time.

Changing the Culture to Support Alertness Management

In order for alertness management strategies to be effective, they must exist in a culture that supports patient and staff safety. Such a culture values proactive responses to patient and staff risks and focuses on systems that can reduce such risks. All the fatigue-reducing efforts in the world will not be effective if such a culture does not exist in an organization. To create a culture that supports alertness management, organizations must identify whether they have a problem with worker fatigue and use a multidisciplinary approach to implement well-considered, appropriate solutions. The organization must also provide visible policy support to those solutions, as well as regular, visible, and consistent endorsement from leadership.

Assessing the Risk

As with any other performance improvement process, before launching an alertness management program, an organization must analyze how its operations, staff, and patients are affected by fatigue. This risk assessment could take many forms, including examining shift lengths and off-duty times and analyzing policies of multiple shifts, overtime, and consecutive duty periods.[1] An organization might want to conduct an anonymous survey to assess the views of staff on fatigue, sleep deprivation, and scheduling. Patient satisfaction surveys can also reveal issues of worker fatigue.

Another source for information about fatigue-related risks is an effective reporting system. This is a system designed to collect information from staff, patients, and organization leadership about actual errors, near misses, or general concerns. Organizations that embody a culture of safety value an effective reporting system because they are as willing to expose areas of weakness as they are to display areas of excellence (*see* Sidebar 2-3 on page 56).[29] Although not all issues reported through a reporting system will relate to fatigue, such a system is a good source of information on fatigue-related events.

To be effective, a fatigue risk assessment should involve a multidisciplinary group so that the issue is examined from a variety of perspectives. Individuals to consider including in such a group include the following:

- Physicians, including representation from the ED, anesthesiology, surgery, radiology, and any other specialty in which members work long hours or rotating shifts

Sidebar 2-3. Reporting Systems

Effective reporting systems are blame free, are easy to use, and elicit a leadership response. Within such a reporting system, all staff members feel that they are supported and safe when voicing concerns. Staff members know they can and are able to speak safely about their own actions or the actions of those in the environment around them, and they are comfortable monitoring others as well.[30]

One way to help staff feel comfortable reporting errors is to call errors by a different name—one that is not as threatening. Terms such as *events*, *blips*, *speed bumps*, and so forth can help reduce the stigma and fear of reporting errors. These terms can refer to both errors that affect patients and near misses.

If staff members find a reporting system difficult to use, they won't use it. To help make reporting easy, it might be helpful to have multiple avenues that staff can take to report concerns. For example, requiring staff to write up a fatigue-related event could be cumbersome, and thus staff might avoid it. Using a one-page form with check boxes might help speed up the process. In addition, an organization might wish to have an "incident hotline" that staff could call any time of day to report any type of event. One organization created a hotline that allowed staff to speak to a live person during the day and leave a message during off hours. The hotline asked the caller for certain details of the event but did not require the caller to leave his or her name.

Data from reporting systems should be tracked and trended. This can help identify problems that could be concealed in day-to-day operations. Problems associated with particular departments, shifts, and times of the year can be discovered by examining in aggregate the issues reported. For example, an organization might discover an elevated number of fatigue-related incidents in the surgery department during the winter. This might indicate a need to look at scheduling or provide more education on fatigue and getting adequate rest.

After analyzing data, organizations should respond to the information generated. This response might include redesigning processes, improving educational efforts, or gathering more information.

As staff members report events, organization leadership must acknowledge these reports and communicate how management addresses the systems responsible for the events. Employee newsletters, staff meetings, posters, and personal contact are all venues through which an organization can acknowledge error reporting.

- Medical students, interns, and residents
- Nurses, including both registered and nonregistered nurses
- Pharmacists
- Administration
- Human resources

To ensure a comprehensive risk assessment, an organization might want to consider using a proactive risk assessment tool, such as failure mode and effects analysis (FMEA), to anticipate problems and see how they could be prevented. FMEA is a team-based, systematic, proactive technique used to prevent process and product problems before they occur. It provides a look not only at what problems could occur but also at how severe the effects of the problems could be. Ideally, FMEA can be used to help prevent failures from occurring. However, if a particular failure cannot be prevented, FMEA then focuses on protections that can be put in place to prevent the failure from reaching the patient, or, in the worst case, to mitigate its effects if it reaches the patient (*see* Sidebar 2-4 below).

Sidebar 2-4. Failure Mode and Effects Analysis (FMEA)

FMEA assumes that no matter how knowledgeable or careful people are, failures will occur in some situations and might even be likely to occur. The focus is on what could allow the failure to occur rather than on whom.

FMEA can involve from as few as 4 to as many as 10 different steps, including the following:

1. Select a high-risk process and assemble a team.
2. Diagram the process and brainstorm potential failure modes.
3. Determine the effects of the failure modes.
4. Prioritize the failure modes.
5. Find root causes of the high-priority failure modes.
6. Redesign the process.
7. Analyze and test the new process.
8. Implement and monitor the redesigned process.

Actions can be identified through FMEA that will reduce the likelihood of error. The product of an FMEA is an action plan that identifies the strategies that the organization intends to implement to prevent or mitigate the effects of a failure.

(continued)

Sidebar 2-4. Failure Mode and Effects Analysis (FMEA) (continued)

The plan should address responsibility for implementation, oversight, pilot testing as appropriate, time lines, and strategies for measuring the effectiveness of the actions.

For fatigue-related issues, a complete FMEA might examine the following aspects of care:

- The use of shifts in providing patient care
- The length of duty periods
- The length of time off between duty periods
- The staffing ratios in high-risk departments, such as surgery, the emergency department, and anesthesiology
- The number of workplace accidents related to fatigue
- The handoff communication strategies in place in the organization

Implementing Fatigue-Related Initiatives

Once an organization has conducted a risk assessment and determined the nature and scope of its fatigue problem, it can begin to address that problem using well-considered approaches, such as the ones outlined earlier in this chapter. Not all strategies will be appropriate for every organization, but a combination of education, alertness strategies, healthy sleep information, and scheduling can help reduce worker fatigue and address problems associated with fatigue. As with other initiatives, organizations should consider using a multidisciplinary approach to implement the initiatives and should involve the staff affected in the design and implementation processes.

It might be helpful for organizations to implement initiatives on a small scale first, such as within a particular department or unit. For example, implementing a planned nap program within the ED or ICU might be beneficial before rolling out the program hospitalwide. Likewise, organizations might want to implement fatigue-reducing strategies targeted to interns and residents before rolling out those strategies to all staff. One effective methodology that can be used to help implement performance initiatives is the plan–do–study–act model. This systematic approach can help ensure positive results on a small scale before a large-scale implementation occurs (*see* Sidebar 2-5 on page 59).

Sidebar 2-5. Plan–Do–Study–Act

Although there are many effective ways to implement an initiative, many organizations use the plan–do–study–act (PDSA) quality improvement technique. Also known as the plan–do–check–act (PDCA) model, the PDSA model emphasizes implementing initiatives on a small scale first and then rolling out to a larger group as success is recognized.

PDSA is a robust performance improvement methodology that works particularly well in health care settings. It is designed to standardize processes and minimize variation, thus eliminating mistakes and rework.

PDSA includes identifying design or redesign opportunities, setting priorities for improvement, and implementing the improvement project. The following are the components of the PDSA cycle.

Plan

- Develop or design a new process or redesign or improve an existing process.
- Determine how to test the new or redesigned process.
- Identify measures that can be used to assess the success of the strategy and whether the objective was reached.
- Determine how to collect the measures of success.
- Involve the right people in the development and testing.

During the planning stage, several issues should be resolved, such as the following:

- Who will be involved in the test?
- What must they know to participate in the test?
- What are the testing timetables?
- How will the test be implemented?
- Why is the idea being tested?
- What are the success factors?
- How will the process and outcomes of the test be measured and assessed?

Do

- Run the test of the new or redesigned process, preferably on a small scale.
- Collect data on the measures of success.

(continued)

Sidebar 2-5. Plan–Do–Study–Act (continued)

Study

- Assess the results of the test.
- Determine whether the change was successful.
- Identify any lessons learned.

Act

- Implement the change permanently.
- Modify it and run it through another testing cycle.
  OR
- Abandon it and develop a new approach to test.

A single initiative can involve a number of different testing phases or different change strategies and can therefore require the use of consecutive PDSA cycles.

Establish Policies That Support an Alertness Management Program

A critical part of implementing an alertness management program is to create policies that support the program. As previously mentioned, if alertness management strategies within an organization are unclear, unsupported, or interpreted as potentially negatively affecting personnel, little progress will be made toward the goal of improving staff sleep and decreasing worker fatigue.[12] However, clear policies that are communicated broadly across an organization and are visibily supported by all levels of leadership in the organization can provide invaluable support for an alertness management program.[12]

Organizations must make sure to distribute these policies and build awareness of them. This can be done by educating staff about the policies, writing about them in corporate newsletters, or introducing them in small-group sessions or staff meetings. As with education on fatigue-related issues, this policy education should not occur just once but should be a continuous process for the organization.

Provide Leadership Support for an Alertness Management Program

Once an alertness management program is in place, it should be reexamined periodically to ensure that it reamins effective. Leaders should be involved in touching base with staff members and making sure they are happy with the program and that the program is doing its job. Walk-arounds—in which leaders visit units and discuss issues with staff—can be a particularly helpful tool in assessing staff satisfaction with a program and determining areas of improvement. A leader's taking the time to talk with staff about the program also signals to the staff that the program

More Information: Addressing Worker Fatigue Not Always Expensive

Addressing sleep deprivation and fatigue might be daunting to some health care organizations that have the perception that significant organizational resources will be needed to design and implement an effective program. However, even if an organization starts small, little changes can make a difference. For example, a brief educational tool shared at staff meetings or during other educational programs does not require a large investment in resources. Likewise, a planned nap program does not have to be cost-prohibitive, and the results of such a program can outweigh the costs. For example, if an organization allows planned naps during long shifts, not only will worker fatigue on the job be reduced, but workers might see the benefits of sleep firsthand, and they might be more likely to respond to the education provided on strategies they personally can implement to reduce fatigue. In some cases, they might change their behavior during their nonwork time, as well as change their behavior during their work time, thus leading to improved performance within the organization.

is important to the organization, and it might reinforce the program. These efforts can go a long way toward establishing a culture thar supports and values the program.

Addressing Doubters

Committing to addressing worker fatigue might be daunting for some organizations, as historical precedents are difficult to change, and long-standing practices—such as having chronically sleep-deprived residents—can be resistant to progress. Some senior physicians who feel they have "paid their dues" might have little sympathy for physicians-in-training and can be resistant to change, especially if they must assume increased responsibility for patient care.[8]

To achieve a culture that supports an alertness management program, an organization must address these naysayers and obtain their buy-in and support. There are a variety of ways to do this, including the following:

- Provide education that specifically addresses their concerns or objections.
- Identify a peer who can serve as a champion for the program. For example, if a well-respected physician endorses a planned nap program and encourages everyone on his or her team to take advantage of it, the program is more likely to gain support and buy-in from other physicians.

- Clearly show the effects of an alertness management program on patient and staff safety.
- Illustrate how such a program has made the the lives of staff—including those of naysayers—better, through improving their sleep opportunities, reducing the risks to their patients, or making their jobs easier.

References

1. Rosekind M.: Managing Fatigue 24/7 in Health Care: Opportunities to Improve Safety. *Anesthesia Patient Safety Foundation Newsletter* vol. 20, Spring 2005. http://www.apsf.org/resource_center/newsletter/2005/spring/06managing.htm (accessed Dec. 1, 2007).

2. Arora V.: Improving the sleep hygiene of medical interns. *Arch Intern Med* 167:1738–1744, Sep. 10, 2007.

3. Wikipedia: *Epworth Sleepiness Scale.* http://en.wikipedia.org/wiki/Epworth_Sleepiness_Scale (accessed Dec. 3, 2007).

4. University of Maryland Medical Center: *Sleep Disorders Center: Sleep-Related Tests & Quizzes: Epworth Sleepiness Scale.* http://www.umm.edu/sleep/epworth_sleep.htm (accessed Dec. 10, 2007).

5. National Sleep Foundation: *Healthy Sleep Tips.* http://www.sleepfoundation.org/site/c.huIXKjM0IxF/b.2417321/k.BAF0/Healthy_Sleep_Tips.htm (accessed Dec. 10, 2007).

6. Caruso C., Condon M.: Night shifts and fatigue. *Am J Nurs* 106:8, Aug. 2006.

7. National Sleep Foundation: *All About Caffeine.* http://www.sleepfoundation.org/site/c.huIXKjM0IxF/b.2465369/apps/nl/content3.asp?content_id=%7B5B9531C4-FAC0-48D9-B46C-B24F705A04CC%7D&notoc=1 (accessed Dec. 3, 2007).

8. Fatigue in healthcare workers. *Healthcare Risk Control. Risk Analysis Employment Issues* 14 (Suppl. A), ECRI, Jan. 2006.

9. National Sleep Foundation: *The Buzz on Caffeine and Sleep.* http://www.sleepfoundation.org/atf/cf/%7BF6BF2668-A1B4-4FE8-8D1A-A5D39340D9CB%7D/caffeine.pdf (accessed Dec. 10, 2007).

10. Gurchiek K.: Study finds eye-opening cost associated with fatigued workers. *HR News,* Jan. 30, 2007.

11. Interview with Vineet Arora, M.D., associate program director for the internal medicine residency at University of Chicago Hospitals, Nov. 19, 2007.

12. Rosekind M.: Managing work schedules: An alertness and safety perspective. In Kryger M., Roth T., Dement W. (eds.): *Principles and Practice of Sleep Medicine*. Philadelphia: Elsevier Science, 2005, pp. 680–690.

13. Gaba D., Howard S.: Fatigue among clinicians and the safety of patients. *N Engl J Med* 347:1249–1274, Oct. 17, 2002.

14. Veasey S., et al.: Sleep loss and fatigue in residency training. *JAMA* 288:1116–1124, Sep. 4, 2002.

15. Arora V., et al.: The effects of on-duty napping on intern sleep time and fatigue. *Ann Intern Med* 144:792–798, 2006.

16. Smith-Coggins R., et al.: Improving alertness and performance in emergency department physicians and nurses: The use of planned naps. *Ann Emerg Med* 48:596–604, Nov. 2006.

17. Rosekind M.R., et al.: Alertness management: Strategic naps in operational settings. *J Sleep Res* 3:62–66, 1995.

18. Interview with Mark Rosekind, Ph.D., president of Alertness Solutions, Nov. 26, 2007.

19. Lockley S., Barger L., Ayas N.: Effects of health care provider work hours and sleep deprivation on safety and performance. *Jt Comm J Qual Patient Saf* 33:7–17, Nov. 2007.

20. National Sleep Foundation: *Most Common Sleep Problems in Women.* http://www.sleepfoundation.org/site/c.huIXKjM0IxF/b.2421125/k.6662/Most_Common_Sleep_Problems_in_Women.htm (accessed Dec. 5, 2007).

21. National Heart Lung and Blood Institute: *What Is Insomnia?* http://www.nhlbi.nih.gov/health/dci/Diseases/inso/inso_whatis.html (accessed Dec. 10, 2007).

22. National Heart Lung and Blood Institute: *What Is Sleep Apnea?* http://www.nhlbi.nih.gov/health/dci/Diseases/SleepApnea/SleepApnea_WhatIs.html (accessed Dec. 3, 2007).

23. National Heart Lung and Blood Institute: *What Is Restless Legs Syndrome?* http://www.nhlbi.nih.gov/health/dci/Diseases/rls/rls_WhatIs.html (accessed Dec. 2, 2007).

24. National Heart Lung and Blood Institute: *What Is Narcolepsy?* http://www.nhlbi.nih.gov/health/dci/Diseases/nar/nar_what.html (accessed Dec. 4, 2007).

25. Blachowicz E., Letizia M.: The challenges of shift work. *Medsurg Nurs* 15:274–280, Oct. 2006.

26. Jha A., Duncan B., Bates D: Fatigue, sleepiness and medical errors. In Shojania K.G., et al. (eds.): *Making Health Care Safer: A Critical Analysis of Patient Safety Practices.* Rockville, MD: Agency for Healthcare Research and Quality, 2001, pp. 519–532.

27. DaRosa D., Bell R.: Four models for surgical resident education under an 80-hour limit. *Surgery* 133: 13–23, Jan. 2003. http://www.acgme.org/acWebsite/dutyHours/dh_McGawSurgery.pdf (accessed Dec. 10, 2007).

28. Parchuram C.: The impact of fatigue on patient safety. *Pediatr Clin North Am* 53:1135–1153, 2006.

29. Marx D.: How building a "just culture" helps an organization learn from errors. *OR Manager* 19:1, 14–15, 20, May 2003.

30. Frankel A.: *Strategies for Building a Hospitalwide Culture of Safety.* Oakbrook Terrace, IL: Joint Commission Resources, 2006.

CHAPTER THREE

Improving Communication to Help Prevent Fatigue-Related Errors

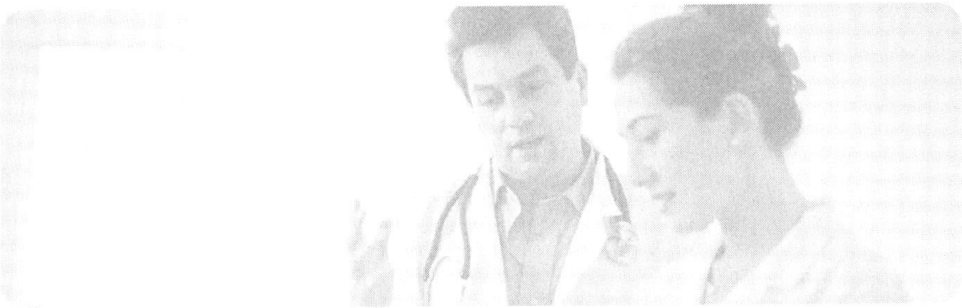

As mentioned in Chapter Two, addressing worker fatigue by implementing strategies that take the health care worker away from the patient—such as reducing work hours, limiting shifts, or scheduling naps—can have unintended consequences, including introducing the risk of poor handoff communication, missed information, and subpar quality of care. Organizations must address these issues when designing an alertness management program to ensure that communication and teamwork are effective, timely, and accurate and that patient care is the best it can possibly be.

Improving Handoff Communication

Handoff communication occurs is when a patient's information and care is "handed off" from one care provider to another. Handoff communication can take place between nurses, physicians, social workers, counselors, and so forth and occurs during shift changes, before and after planned naps, and at any other time care is transferred from one staff person to another. Effective communication during handoffs is critical because if information is not timely, complete, and accurate, mistakes can be made, options can be overlooked, and patient care can be comprised. Consider the example of a patient who was receiving treatment for chest pains and who was also on antidepressant medication. During the patient's initial assessment, the nurse performing the assessment determined that the patient was at low risk for suicide but should be watched and reassessed throughout his stay. Because of an incomplete handoff communication, the information about the antidepressant medication and suicide potential was not shared, and the nurse assuming the patient's care was not aware of the potential danger. The patient's heart condition took a turn for the worse, and the patient reacted poorly. He attempted suicide while the nurse was out of the room. Had the handoff communication been more thorough, the nurse assuming the patient's care could have been more prepared, and the situation possibly could have been avoided.

There are a variety of ways to ensure effective handoff communication. Following are some points to keep in mind regarding effective handoff communication.

Keep the interaction concise and accurate. What a staff member includes in handoff communication varies by setting and discipline but can include a summary of the patient's current medical status, resuscitation status, recent lab values, and allergies, along with a problem list and a to-do list for the covering physician or nurse.

Use clear language. Staff should avoid unclear or potentially confusing terms ("she's a little unstable," "he's doing fine," or "she's lethargic") in handoff communications. Instead, staff should be as specific as possible. For example, it might be prudent to share the patient's current blood pressure, heart rate, and other vital signs to help provide a picture of the patient's condition to oncoming staff. Staff members also should not use abbreviations or jargon that could be misinterpreted.

Incorporate effective communication techniques. These techniques could include limiting interruptions, focusing on the information being exchanged, and allocating sufficient time for the communication exchange. Implementing read-back or check-back techniques to make sure there is a common understanding about expectations can be helpful (*see* Sidebar 3-1, above). Encouraging interactive questioning to allow for better information absorption is also beneficial. Staff

Sidebar 3-1. Tools That Help with Handoff Communication

The following are some specific tools organizations might find helpful in structuring handoff communications:

- **"At-a-glance"** summary: An at-a-glance summary uses paper forms or visual displays that make it easy for all health care workers to access information, thereby reducing the need to include the information from the summary in the handoff.
- **Shift handoff checklist:** A checklist can be filled out by the outgoing shift for each handoff. Not only does it offer a standard set of cues to help staff members remember important information, it also provides a history to which other staff members can refer.
- **Computerized handoff:** Computerized handoff forms can provide the same cues as checklists and summaries, and they also allow the information to be included in the patient's electronic medical record. Using this computerized form makes a patient's information accessible to all staff involved in the patient's care.

Sidebar 3-2. Situation–Background–Assessment–Recommendation (SBAR)

The Situation–Background–Assessment–Recommendation (SBAR) technique is an easy-to-remember, concrete mechanism that is useful for framing any conversation, especially critical ones, requiring a clinician's immediate attention and action. The technique can be used to standardize the type of information shared between individuals and helps set the expectation that specific informational elements are going to be communicated every time a patient is discussed. The SBAR technique can be useful during handoff communications to convey information quickly, concisely, and completely. SBAR involves the following steps:

- **Situation:** This is the part of the technique in which the two parties communicating establish the topic about which they are going to speak. For example, if engaging in a handoff communication, the parties should share their names, the patient's name, and the patient's room number. If there is a specific problem to discuss, the clinician handing off the patient should briefly state the problem, when it happened or started, and how severe it is.

- **Background:** The clinician handing off care should provide relative background information on the patient being handed off, including the following, when appropriate:
    - Admitting diagnosis and date of admission
    - List of current medications, allergies, intravenous fluids, and labs
    - Most recent vital signs
    - Lab results, with the date and time a test was performed and results of previous tests for comparison
    - Other clinical information
    - Code status

- **Assessment:** The clinician should state his or her assessment of the situation and the patient's status.

- **Recommendation:** The clinician should offer a recommendation of what to do next. For example, if there are specific instructions related to the patient, the clinician might want to share them at this time.

should keep patient reports patient centered and avoid irrelevant details. One specific tool organizations can use to structure handoff communications is the Situation–Background–Assesment–Recommendation (SBAR) tool (*see* Sidebar 3-2, above).

Standardize communications. Using a consistent format for handoff communication can increase the amount of information staff members accurately record and

More Information: Repeat-Back

Repeat-back is a closed-loop communication tool that helps improve the reliability of an information exchange between two or more people.[3] The tool involves four distinct actions:

1. The "sender" concisely states information to the "receiver."
2. The receiver repeats back what he or she heard.
3. The sender acknowledges that the repeat-back was correct or makes a correction.
4. The process continues until a shared understanding is verified. Within this model, responding to a message with an "okay" or an "uh-huh" is not sufficient to close the communication loop. The message must be explicitly restated and acknowledged.

Organizations can use this type of closed-loop communication during handoff communications to help smooth the communication process and ensure that no critical information is lost. If team members practice this type of communication during routine circumstances, they will be well prepared to use it during acute instances when time pressure and urgency are factors.[13]

recall and can improve their ability to plan patient care. Organizations might want to consider organizing patient data within handoff communications with a sign-out checklist, a script, or an "at-a-glance" status display. These can provide cues of important information to pass on that is otherwise likely to be forgotten in the chaos of shift or personnel changes.

Use technology. Communication systems that transmit information across settings and care providers bring consistency and coordination to care practices. For example, automated medication reconciliation between settings of care, such as physician office practices and a hospital, streamlines and increases safety during admissions and discharges. In addition, electronic medical records can facilitate transitions by providing consistent, accessible information about patients and their care. Staff members should be able to readily access essential components of care, such as whether a newly ordered medication was administered, whether labs were done, or whether a do-not-resuscitate order is in place. Technology can also be used to sign off patient care. For example, a large teaching hospital in the Northwest uses a computerized sign-out system, which automatically updates a patient's drug allergies, current medications, results of recent tests, relevant medical history, and code status. Interns enter daily updates on their patients' current conditions and basic treatment plans. This information is available to all nursing and physician staff groups.[1] Staff members should keep electronic approaches interactive and effective by making time to answer questions or provide updates before signing off responsibility.

Involving Patients in Handoff Communication

Patients and families can and should be involved in ensuring effective handoff communication, as they are in a position to let nurses and physicians know when something has changed in their condition or care. As part of involving patients in handoff communication, patients and their families should be empowered to speak up and let their health care providers know if something is worrisome or has changed. If staff communicate effectively and frequently with the patient and family, the patient is more involved in his or her care and can help identify potential errors and help with continuity between care providers (*see* Sidebar 3-3 on page 71).

It can be helpful for health care workers to touch base with patients sometime before, during, or after a handoff. At some point, a physician or nurse might want to converse with a patient about who will be taking up the patient's care after that caregiver has left. This can be done through a variety of means, including telling the patient about the new physician or nurse, writing his or her name on the wipe board in the patient's room, or showing the patient a picture of the oncoming physician or nurse. By keeping the patient in the loop about who is picking up his or her care, physicians and nurses can empower patients to be involved in their care.

More Information: Fostering Communication with Patients

Organizations that value patient safety and involvement in care have programs and structures in place to help foster open communication with the patient and family. There are many such programs and structures, but the scope of this publication does not allow an in-depth discussion. This box offers a brief discussion of some valuable programs to improve patient–staff communication. More information can be found in *The Joint Commission Guide to Patient and Family Education*.

- Require education for physicians, nurses, and other clinical staff that addresses the importance of including the patient in his or her care. Such education programs should also provide tips on how to communicate effectively with patients. Staff should be taught to do the following:
  - Involve patients in their care.
  - Encourage questions.
  - Prompt full answers to questions, not just "yes" or "no."
  - Be explicit in patient care instructions.

(continued)

More Information: Fostering Communication with Patients (continued)

- Actively listen to patients.
- Observe and interpret body language.
- Use terminology that is easy to understand.

Physicians, in particular, need focused training on how to effectively communicate with patients. Medical schools do not typically teach listening skills or encourage physicians to empathize with their patients. Organizations might need to overcome the educational experiences of physicians in order to improve patient–physician dynamics. In order to elicit physician participation, an organization might have to emphasize the benefits of good patient–physician communication. Not only can patient outcomes be positively affected, but poor physician communication styles have been linked to the risk of malpractice litigation.[4]

- Educate patients on how they can be involved in their own care. This can include encouraging patients to speak up when they have questions or concerns and to use health care professionals as sources of information on conditions and treatment options. The Joint Commission has several tools that can be used to help empower patients to participate in their own care. (*See* Sidebar 3-3 on page 71 for an example.)

- Provide patients access to multidisciplinary teams. The multidisciplinary rounds process brings many different disciplines together for a daily meeting with the patient and his or her family. During this meeting, the group discusses treatment options, plans, and concerns. Group rounds not only involve patients in their care but provide an opportunity for enhanced communication between staff and patients. Such rounds can also help with continuity of care as patients and their treatment teams have a designated time and space in which to discuss care.

- Use effective tools for communication. Many individuals in the United States cannot read above a fifth-grade level. Organizations should design written materials for patients to be easy to read and understand. In addition to printed materials, organizations might wish to use other tools to improve communication with patients. For example, wipe boards can be used in a patient's room or wherever else information needs to be communicated between staff and patients. These boards provide a place where staff can list the names of the physician, nurse, and other staff treating the patient. The boards can also provide a place for family members to write questions to ask the physician or nurse when he or she next visits.[5]

Sidebar 3-3. The Joint Commission's Speak Up Campaign

The following are the components of The Joint Commission's Speak Up campaign, whose goal is to get patients more involved in their own care:

- **S**peak up if you have questions or concerns, and if you don't understand, ask again. It's your body, and you have a right to know.
- **P**ay attention to the care you are receiving. Make sure you're getting the right treatments and medications from the right health care professionals. Don't assume anything.
- **E**ducate yourself about your diagnosis, the medical tests you are undergoing, and your treatment plan.
- **A**sk a trusted family member or friend to be your advocate.
- **K**now what medications you take and why you take them. Medication errors are the most common health care errors.
- **U**se a hospital, clinic, surgery center, or other type of health care organization that has undergone a rigorous on-site evaluation against established state-of-the-art quality and safety standards, such as that provided by the Joint Commission.
- **P**articipate in all decisions about your treatment. You are the center of the health care team.

Other Speak Up initiatives from the Joint Commission include the following:

- ***Help Prevent Errors in Your Care: For Surgical Patients*** includes tips to help patients prepare for surgery and make sure they have the correct procedure performed at the correct site on their body.
- ***Three Things You Can Do to Prevent Infection*** highlights three easy things everyone can do to prevent infection and help avoid contagious diseases such as the common cold, strep throat, and influenza.
- ***Things You Can Do to Prevent Medication Mistakes*** presents valuable information about preventing medication mistakes as well as helpful questions to ask a physician, pharmacist, nurse, or other caregiver at the clinic, hospital, physicians' office, or pharmacy. The brochure includes a detachable wallet card for listing medications. This campaign was developed at

(continued)

Sidebar 3-3. The Joint Commission's Speak Up Campaign (continued)

the urging of employers who asked the Joint Commission for patient safety materials they could provide to their employees.

All materials for the Speak Up campaign are available on the Joint Commission Web site, at http://www.jointcommission.org.

Case Study 3-1.
Pella Regional Health Center

For several years, the nursing staff within the medical/surgical (med/surg) unit at Pella Regional Health Center—a private, nonprofit, 25-bed rural critical access hospital located in Pella, Iowa—had a process for communicating information at shift change; however, nurses within the unit had concerns about how long this process took and the quality of information shared during this time. In August 2006, the med/surg unit began reviewing its nursing change-of-shift report process, using methods gained from a course in Lean methodology to revise the process and address nurses' concerns.[6]

What Is Lean Methodology?

Lean methodology is an industrial philosophy long embraced by manufacturing innovators such as Toyota Motor Corporation. It involves determining the value of different steps in any given process and eliminating waste. The ultimate goal of the methodology is to design a process in which every step adds value.[7]

Three nurses from the med/surg unit who had been trained in Lean used this methodology to revise change-of-shift communication. In the initial phases of the revision process, the nurses held a preconceived opinion that simply moving to a taped change-of-shift report would effectively address nursing needs. "However, after looking at the process using the Lean methodology, the nurses determined that the quality of the information being shared was the primary issue," says Janet Naset-Payne, director of inpatient services for Pella Regional Health Center.

To improve the quality of information shared during this critical nursing communication time, the three nurses created an outline of items to be discussed during an effective handoff. The nurses invited Naset-Payne to participate in developing this outline, to assist in adding patient safety concerns and quality indicators into the outline as well as clinical issues. "Having the bedside nurses develop the outline was critical to its success, and the additional emphasis on patient safety and quality indicators brought a much broader perspective to the project and gave great depth to the tool," says Naset-Payne.

When developing the outline, the group formatted it using the following acronym:

I: Identify (patient demographics)
N: Needs (patient care)
F: Fall/suicide/skin risks
O: Orders received on shift
R: Results (abnormal only)
M: Medications (including medication reconciliation)

Within each lettered category, several questions prompt the user to share appropriate information. Some information prompted by the tool includes the admitting diagnosis and symptoms, pain interventions, risk assessments, and abnormal vital signs (*see* Figure 3-1 below).

Figure 3-1.
Nurse-to-Staff Report

Pella Regional Health Center

Nurse to Staff Report
INFORM

Identify, Patient Demographics

- Pt. Name / Age / Room No. / Level of Care
- Admission Date / Time
- Admitting Diagnosis / Symptoms / Physician
- Allergies / Adverse Reactions
- Isolation Precautions
- Living Arrangements / ADLs
- Code Status

Needs, Patient Care

- IV Status – site, volume up
- Respiratory Therapy – oxygen, treatments
- Foley Catheter / NG / Other Drains – output, appearance

(continued)

Figure 3-1. (continued)
Nurse-to-Staff Report

- PT / OT / ST / Massage Therapy
- Pain Access / Intervention
- Concerns – treatment, safety
- Education

Fall / Suicide / Skin Risks
- Fall Levels (Min, Mod, Max)
- Suicide (High, No Risk)
- Skin (High, No Risk)
- Other Risks Identified

Orders
- Received on your shift

Results
- (**Abnormal Only**) Assessment, Test / Study Results
- Physician Notification
- Pending Tests / Studies

Medications
- Flu and Pneumonia vaccine
- Changes / Effectiveness
- Medication Reconciliation – completed / follow-up needed
- Other Medication Management Information

Source: Pella Regional Health Care, Pella, Iowa. Used with permission.

This figure outlines Pella Regional Health Center's INFORM tool used during handoff communications.

The Revised Shift Change Report

Using the INFORM tool, the three nurses revised the change-of-shift report process as follows. Just before a change of shift, each med/surg nurse enters the report room and tapes his or her shift report. The report room is a designated quiet room on the unit where there is a tape recorder and a laminated copy of the INFORM tool. The nurse uses the INFORM tool as a guide to the shift report's content. The tool is not a checklist, nor is it included in the patient's medical record. It is a tool that nurses can use to frame their handoff communication. Nurses do their reporting one at a time so patient care is not interrupted.

Nurses beginning their shift listen to all recorded nursing reports from the previous shift. After completing this task, each nurse meets one-on-one with the nurse he or she is relieving. During this session, the two nurses can ask questions, clarify information, and review orders together. This revised change-of-shift process allows for streamlined communication of important clinical, safety, and quality-of-care information.

Educating Staff on the New Process

Once the new change-of-shift process was designed, the three nurses educated nursing staff on the med/surg unit. They presented the new process during staff meetings and developed posters describing the process that were hung throughout the unit. The new process began in 2006. During implementation, the three nurses listened in on change-of-shift report tapings, worked with staff as needed, and continually served as mentors for the process.

Measuring Success

To measure the success of the new change-of-shift report, Pella Regional Health Center looked at a variety of data. "We compared data on falls to see if the new communication process helped reduce patient falls," says Naset-Payne. "Our fall rate dropped 32% between fourth quarter 2006 and first quarter 2007." The organization also looked at core measure data on discharge education and found that after the new change-of-shift report process was in place, there was 100% compliance with discharge teaching, maintaining the score from the third quarter. Previous scores on this core measure were in the 50% range.

"We also wanted feedback from the nurses on the new process, so we conducted a survey three months after implementation. The results showed that 87% of med/surg nurses felt information shared during the report was important to the care of the patient. Nurses also felt they are leaving the shift in a timelier manner," says Naset-Payne. The popularity of the INFORM tool grew "as [obtetric (OB)] nurses floated to the med/surg unit and were able to experience its positive impact, which resulted in a request to use the tool in their area. This was a real testament to the effectiveness and usefulness of the tool," says Naset-Payne.

Rolling Out the Tool Housewide

The INFORM tool has been so successful in the med/surg unit that the organization is rolling out the tool to all departments within the hospital. "We are using the INFORM tool as a template, and each department is individualizing the tool to fit the needs of its area. Initially we asked departments not to alter the outline, only highlight information important to their area. Since this time we have allowed specialty areas such as OB to change it and make it more specific to their area, still using the acronym INFORM," says Ronda Reimer, R.N., special projects coordinator for Pella Regional Health Center (*see* Figure 3-2, below). Ultimately, the organization hopes to use the INFORM tool during every patient transfer or staff shift change within the organization. "We are even involving physicians in the process and are working with them to use the INFORM tool when communicating with other physicians covering their patients," says Reimer.

Figure 3-2.
Obstetric (OB) Nurse-to-Staff Report

Pella Regional Health Center

Nurse to Staff Report
INFORM - OB

Identify, Patient Demographics

- Pt Name / Room No.
- Age
- Gravida / Para
- EDC / Adm Date / Del'd Date & Time
- Physician
- Husband / Significant Other Name
- Blood Type / Rubella / GBS
- Social History

Needs, Patient Care

- IV Status / Charges
- Education
- Stork – paper work
- Delivery Type and Perineum / Incision Care
- Breastfeeding – needs
- Antibiotics – medications / time/ reason
- Intrathecal – Epidural Time / SL

Fundus / Fall / Suicide

- Location

Figure 3-2. (continued)
Obstetric (OB) Nurse-to-Staff Report

- Consistency
- Bleeding
- Medication – if necessary
- Suicide Risks
- Fall Risk Level – Due to void-tolerating activity

Orders
- Received on your shift

Results
- (**Abnormal ONLY**) Assessment, Test / Study Results
- Physician Notifications
- Pending Tests / Studies

Medications
- Changes During Shift
- Last time given
- Rhogham / MMR Given
- Medication Reconciliation – completed / follow-up needed

Source: Pella Regional Health Care, Pella, Iowa. Used with permission.

Pella Regional Health Care uses this tool to streamline communications within the OB department.

One of the keys to successful implementation of the INFORM tool housewide is allowing each department to individualize the tool for its own use. "How the nuclear medicine department uses the INFORM tool, for example, is going to be different from how the med/surg unit uses it. Allowing departments to make the tool fit their dynamics helps generate buy-in and support," says Reimer.

Within the organization's mock tracer process, individuals conducting the tracer verify how the INFORM tool is being used during handoff communications. "The INFORM tool can be repeatedly encountered as you follow a patient through the care continuum. Staff members throughout the hospital are starting to use INFORM as an outline for any handoff communication," says Naset-Payne.

By streamlining the handoff communication process and ensuring the quality of information communicated during handoffs, Pella Regional Health Center is improving communication during shift changes, during patient transfers, at discharge, and at other critical times throughout the care continuum.

Fostering Teamwork

In addition to improving handoff communication, organizations can address the potentially negative consequences of multiple caregivers treating the same patient by fostering a team environment. By changing the mind-set from one individual caring for the patient throughout his or her continuum of care to a mind-set of teamwork, collaboration, and individuals working together to provide the safest and most appropriate care, organizations can reap the benefits of both reducing fatigue and increasing teamwork. Instead of placing sole responsibility for a patient's care on a team member who is possibly fatigued, the patient care team can work together to care for the patient, thus allowing the fatigued team member to take a planned nap or leave his or her shift.

Unfortunately, health care providers, particularly physicians, are trained to think as individuals rather than as team members. In order to improve staff communication and teamwork, an organization might need to overcome the individual-focused perspectives of its staff and licensed independent practitioners.

Effective teams have defined and measurable goals, a clear division of labor, and effective systems that support them. They are characterized by trust, respect, and collaboration. Effective teams regularly participate in team-training activities, and they have an open and honest flow of communication. Team members value familiarity over formality and watch out for each other to make sure mistakes aren't made.

In order to emphasize the importance of teamwork and communication, an organization should take the following actions:

- Eliminate hierarchy.
- Delineate team members' roles and responsibilities.
- Use effective communication techniques.
- Provide training on teamwork and effective communication.
- Measure team performance.
- Enforce a zero-tolerance policy for abusive behavior.

Eliminating Hierarchy

Effective teams do not allow hierarchy to be present. Hierarchy is the antithesis of a team. When hierarchy differences exist, people on the lower end of the hierarchy tend to be uncomfortable, if not downright afraid, about speaking up about problems or concerns. Gruff, aggressive, or intimidating behavior by individuals at the top of a hierarchy can stifle communication and give the impression that these individuals are unapproachable.

Conversely, individuals on the higher end of the hierarchy may think that concerns brought up by others are unwarranted or challenging to their authority. Consider a nurse who watches a physician, who is covering for a napping colleague, prescribe a medication for a patient that the colleague noted was incompatible with a current medication the patient is taking. The nurse desperately wants to say something, but the physician has a history of not reacting well to criticism. The nurse keeps quiet and changes the medication later, against the physician's orders. The patient is not harmed, but the potential for teamwork and appropriate care is lost.

Organizations that want to eliminate hierarchy in health care workers must set the tone across the organization. Organization leadership must encourage collaboration, respect the input of all the staff, and accept nothing less than team performance.

Physicians, in particular, should be encouraged to eliminate hierarchies. Many times, physicians aren't aware of hierarchies that exist between them and other staff members because they are usually at the top of any hierarchy. Often, physicians perceive the health care environment as collaborative when it really isn't. Providing feedback to physicians on their communication abilities and any perceived hierarchies can be helpful in alerting them to potential problems and empowering them to change.

Although effective teams do not have a hierarchy, they do have a leader. This might seem like a subtle difference, but it is a very distinct one. A team leader sets the tone for team interactions. He or she works to flatten hierarchies by using first names, engaging team members in the care process, and incorporating the suggestions and expertise of individual team members into the clinical plan.[9]

Delineating Roles and Responsibilities

Effective teams are made up of individuals who are aware of the roles they play in the team as well as the roles other team members play. Confusion about roles and responsibilities can cause communication failures, as individuals don't know what they are supposed to do and how they are supposed to interact with others. Clearly delineating the roles and responsibilities of each team member makes everyone aware of the part they play in the whole and helps them contribute and communicate information necessary for appropriate patient care.

Using Effective Communication Techniques

A hallmark of a good team is the effectiveness of its communication. To help foster communication, organizations might want to consider using some of the following communication techniques within their patient care teams:

- **Briefings:** Briefings are short discussions between team members that aim to get all clinicians at a common beginning. Briefings can help promote a sense

More Information: Looking to Aviation for Answers

There are a variety of ways organizations can encourage a team approach to care. As no organization has time to reinvent the wheel, it might be helpful to look to other industries, such as aviation, for examples of how to encourage teamwork and communication.

In the late 1970s, the aviation industry began addressing teamwork and communication among its flight crews. The industry discovered that within these crews, hierarchies existed, individuals felt uncomfortable challenging pilots, and interactive communication was almost nonexistent. In many ways, the crew of a large aircraft is similar to a patient care team in a hospital. Historically, the pilot, like the physician, assumed absolute control and did not take kindly to questions about his or her decisions.

To overcome communication problems, the aviation industry developed a training program that added teamwork skills to the traditionally taught technical skills. Crew resource management (CRM), now widely used by airlines, helps teach a flight crew how to draw upon the different capabilities and knowledge of a given crew. Assertiveness training, adaptability, leadership, and decision making are all taught as a part of the program. Crew members engage in simulation exercises, role-playing exercises, and self-critiques to practice effective communication techniques. Interactive group debriefings are also used to help improve communication.[11]

of collaboration between team members, set the tone for open communication, and bring everyone onto the same page to avoid surprises. During briefings, a patient care team gathers to compare notes, identify what they want to accomplish, identify resources, and anticipate obstacles.[10] Successful briefings are structured and quick. They involve all team members. Individuals conducting a briefing should use first names and make eye contact with other team members. This establishes a tone of collaboration and encourages individuals to speak up.[9]

- **Debriefings:** Whereas briefings can be helpful before a procedure, debriefings can be helpful when a process had ended. They allow team members to discuss how things went, outcomes, opportunities for improvement, and elements of success. Debriefings allow a team to better prepare for the next encounter and avoid repeating the same mistakes.
- **Call-out:** This communication technique requires team members to call out each phase of a process as they are entering it so that all team members know

to proceed. When using the call-out technique, participants should speak clearly and loudly so all team members can hear.[10]

Providing Team Training

Telling health care professionals to "act as a team" will achieve few, if any, results. An important step in creating effective teams is to provide team training to all staff members that teaches them how to be part of an effective team. Without training, teams are just diverse groups of people that work side by side. Training can mold a group into a unified entity that can face problems, identify issues, and work together to care for a patient.

During team training, organizations should emphasize the value of teamwork and the potential results of effective teamwork and should also provide staff members with training on critical tools and behaviors that can help enhance teamwork. The following sections discuss some important tools and behaviors that relate to effective communication and teamwork.

Assertiveness Training

Although the presence of hierarchies can intimidate individuals and prevent them from speaking up about concerns or problems, hierarchy is not the only reason people do not speak up. Sometimes individuals don't feel comfortable sharing bad news or asserting themselves. Assertiveness training can be helpful in providing tips and strategies for individuals who have difficulty speaking up. It can provide a framework that individuals can use to communicate about concerns or problems. In many organizations, assertiveness training is appropriate for nurses and other staff who work with physicians.

When a person asserts himself or herself, the individual should be pleasant yet persistent. Being assertive does not mean being aggressive, hostile, or confrontational. There are five elements to making an assertive statement:

1. Get the individual's attention.
2. State the concern.
3. State the problem.
4. Offer a solution.
5. Obtain agreement.[10]

In some cases, providing individuals with an assertiveness checklist can be helpful. This is a list of things that individuals can do to effectively and positively assert themselves so their opinions are heard.

In addition to educating staff members on assertiveness, it is important to offer training on how to react to assertive statements. If someone makes an assertive statement and it is unfounded, it is important not to squelch the person's input but to use it as a teaching opportunity. This type of training is particularly important for physicians because physicians will potentially not react well to assertive statements from other staff members due to perceived hierarchies.

Conflict Resolution

Many times health care staff would rather work around a problem than discuss it. This not only works against team behavior, but it can also set up scenarios where errors can occur. For example, consider a nurse who would rather risk a potential medical error than confront a physician with the fact that he overlooked a key element of a patient's care because he was tired.

Effective teams know how to deal with conflict and resolve it, if possible. Training and education on conflict resolution is necessary for team survival. Staff should be taught to discuss conflicts in a respectful yet firm manner. Teaching staff to use phrases such as "I perceive an issue here" or "It seems to me that..." can be helpful. Teams can be trained on structured communication methods that can help resolve conflicts before they get out of hand. An example of such a structured communication method is the "two-attempt rule." With this method, if a person has a concern and assertively states that concern but there is no response from the team or the individual to whom the concern is expressed, then the person with the concern or another team member can assert the concern a second time in the same manner. If a response is still not given, and there is a concern about patient safety, the person with the concern is responsible for taking the concern up the chain of command to the supervisor (*see* Sidebar 3-4 below).[10] This report should be received without judgment or blame, and the individual reporting should not be chastised.

Sidebar 3-4. A Chain-of-Command Policy

It is often difficult for a health care worker to challenge a physician. There are times, however, when challenging physician orders is appropriate, and even necessary, to prevent errors. Organization leaders might want to establish a chain-of-command policy to help staff feel more comfortable questioning things. A chain-of-command policy is a formal administrative tool that provides employees with a process to resolve administrative, clinical, or other patient safety or service issues. Employees can use a chain-of-command policy and procedures to present an issue of concern and pass it up the lines of authority until it is resolved.[12] All staff members should be trained on the policy and assured that invoking it will not be held against them.

How to Conduct Teamwork Training

Despite the importance of teamwork and effective communication training, many organizations do not engage in this activity. As one expert put it, "It is ironic indeed to realize that a football team spends 40 hours a week practicing teamwork for the 2 hours on Sunday afternoon when their teamwork really counts. Teams in organizations seldom spend 2 hours per year practicing when their ability to function as a team counts 40 hours per week"—and often more for health care teams.[13]

Teamwork training might involve bringing together groups of health care providers to get to know each other, engage in team-building exercises, talk frankly about current communication issues, and work together to solve communication problems. A complicating factor for health care teams is that team members are continually changing. This is one of the reasons that true teamwork can be difficult to achieve in health care organizations.

Team training can also involve role-playing exercises. As mentioned previously, physicians many times aren't aware of the hierarchies that exist between them and other staff members. They might perceive the health care environment as collaborative when it really isn't. Role-playing exercises can build awareness of one's own communication patterns and provide structured opportunities for the practice and critique of new behaviors.[14]

Team training for staff members can be enhanced by storytelling because it teaches others about mistakes and successes. Organizations should encourage staff members to share their stories so that everyone can learn from them. Almost every health care worker has a story of how fatigue and sleep deprivation affected his or her ability to provide care. By sharing these stories, teams can see how common the issue is and potentially learn from others' experiences.

Involving Physicians in Teamwork Training

As previously mentioned, in most organizations, physicians are at the top of any perceived hierarchy. Because of the high-profile nature of their positions, physicians must support, endorse, and actively participate in team training and team building in order for successful team-based care to take place. Physicians on staff at an organization, as well as those who have privileges in that organization but who are not on staff, should be involved in any team-training exercises. Organizations might want to identify some champions within the physician community who can actively promote, support, and participate in the process of team training. Peer pressure can be a very good motivator in encouraging other physicians to be part of a team.

Training, Training, and Training Again

Teamwork is not learned overnight. It requires constant practice and regular reinforcement. Team training should be an ongoing exercise in an organization. New staff, new procedures, and changing environments all require constant reinforcement of the team mentality. Even staff members who have received previous team training can benefit from a refresher course. Just like a football team, a health care team should be constantly trained on how to effectively operate and communicate.

Measuring Team Performance

Measuring team performance allows an organization to determine whether teams are functioning effectively and whether training and education efforts have been adequate and appropriate. Measurement results can show that teams are functioning well and also help indicate the need for further work toward a team-based approach to care. Some metrics or benchmarks to consider when measuring team performance include the following:

- The number of adverse events
- The number of disruptive behavior episodes
- Staff satisfaction
- Patient satisfaction
- Staffing changes

There are a variety of ways to collect data on these metrics and benchmarks, including patient and staff surveys, observation, reporting systems, focus groups, and so forth. As with all other data collection, what an organization does with its team performance data is critical. Organizations should use data to identify areas of success as well as areas of improvement, to work on any problem areas that arise, and to provide feedback to team members.

Enforcing a Zero-Tolerance Policy Toward Anti-Team Behavior

Despite an organization's emphasis on teamwork and effective communication, some individuals might not buy into the concept of teamwork. Or, some individuals might not be able to control their anger and use an effective communication technique. Individuals such as these might still exhibit aggressive or intimidating behavior. They might not allow questions, might shut down collaboration, and might ignore input. If an organization's leadership does not enforce a zero-tolerance policy for this type of behavior, then all the team training in the world will be for naught. If staff feel that leadership will overlook abusive and intimidating behavior, then the motivation for team behavior is greatly reduced. Communication between team members can be stifled, and the organization is back where it began. Talking about teamwork and effective communication is not enough. Both physicians and staff must realize that teamwork and effective communication are required by the organization, and intimidation and power struggles will not be tolerated. For individuals struggling with how to effectively communicate, personal coaching or mentoring might be helpful because it gives the individuals someone with whom they can directly work to improve their skills.

Conclusion

Patient care is safest and most effective when it is provided by a team whose members effectively communicate with one another. Problems associated with fatigue can be mitigated when team members support each other and work together to provide care. Effective communication and teamwork are critical elements to improving patient safety and reducing the negative effects of fatigue.

References

1. Volpp K.G., Grande D.: Residents' suggestions for reducing errors in teaching hospitals. *N Engl J Med* 348:851–855, Feb. 27, 2003.

2. Institute for Healthcare Improvement: *SBAR Technique for Communication: A Situational Briefing Model.* http://www.ihi.org/IHI/Topics/PatientSafety/SafetyGeneral/Tools/SBARTechniqueforCommunicationASituationalBriefingModel.htm (accessed Dec. 15, 2007).

3. Mound T.: Closing the communication loop: Using read-back/hear-back to support patient safety. *Jt Comm J Qual Patient Saf* 30:460–464, Aug. 2004.

4. Levinson W., et al.: Physician–patient communication: The relationship with malpractice claims among primary care physicians and surgeons. *JAMA* 277:553–557, 1997.

5. Edgman-Levitan S.: Involving the patient in safety efforts. In Leonard M., Frankel A., Simmonds T.: *Achieving Safe and Reliable Healthcare.* Chicago: Heath Administration Press, 2004.

6. Healthcare Performance Partners reVIEW© Realizing Exceptional Value In Everyday Work, Cindy Jimmerson with contributions by Durward Sobek. ©Cindy Jimmerson, 2004. http://leanhealthcareperformance.com/leanhealthcare/leanhealthcare-services.php (accessed Dec. 15, 2007).

7. Institute for Healthcare Improvement: *Going Lean in Healthcare*, 2005. http://www.ihi.org/NR/rdonlyres/F4E4084A-6297-44DB-8A78-75008F6DA7A1/0/GoingLeaninHealthCareWhitePaper.pdf (accessed Dec. 10, 2007).

8. Grumbach K., Bodenheimer T.: Can health care teams improve primary care practice? *JAMA* 291:1246–1251, Mar. 10, 2004.

9. Leonard M., Frankel A., Simmonds T.: *Achieving Safe and Reliable Healthcare.* Chicago: Heath Administration Press, 2004.

10. Air Force's 11 patient safety tools build better team communication. *OR Manager* 19:1, 12–13, Feb. 2003.

11. Bianchi-Sand S.: It takes a team to prevent errors. *Am J Nurs* 103:89–90, Dec. 2003.

12. Jones J.S.: Chain of command: A risk management perspective. *Compass: Navigating Today's Healthcare Risks & Liabilities* 2:1–4, Mar. 2004.

13. Wise H., et al.: *Making Health Teams Work.* Cambridge, MA: Ballinger Publishing Company, 1974.

14. Farbstein K.: Role-playing case simulations: A tool to improve communication and enhance safety. *Jt Comm J Qual Patient Saf* 29:261, May 2003.

CHAPTER FOUR

Preventing Worker Burnout

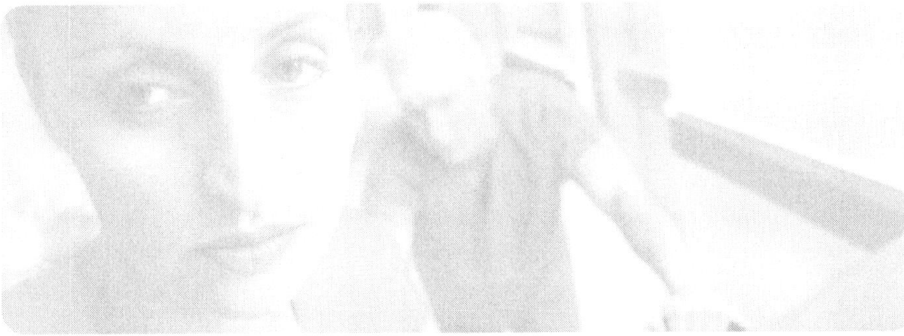

One often hears people say, "I am so burned out," or, "My work is burning me out," but what does *burnout* really mean? Burnout is a relatively new term in the English language—coined in the 1970s to describe situations akin to a nervous breakdown or depression.[1] According to one definition, *burnout* is a psychological term describing the experience of long-term exhaustion and diminished interest, usually in the work context. It is often construed as a result of a period of expending too much effort at work while having too little recovery.[2] Burnout has also been described as the end result of stress that combines emotional exhaustion, depersonalization, and low personal accomplishment.[3] Christina Maslach, Ph.D., an expert in worker burnout, described the concept as "a syndrome of physical and emotional exhaustion involving the development of negative job attitudes and perception, a poor professional self-concept, and a loss of empathy and concern for the client being serviced.[4]

When an individual is burned out at work, day-to-day challenges can seem insurmountable, the work environment and everyone in it can appear bleak, and the individual often has difficultly mustering the energy to care.

Who Is Subject to Burnout?

Cordes and Doherty found that workers who have frequent intense or emotionally charged interactions with others are especially susceptible to burnout.[5] High-stress jobs can lead to more burnout than low-stress ones, and consequently health care workers are often prone to burnout.

Physicians can be particularly subject to burnout. The practice of medicine is increasingly more competitive, and reimbursement from most insurance companies does not favor physicians. Patient expectations coupled with the threat of law suits and the cost of malpractice insurance contribute to a situation in which many physicians are frustrated, dissatisfied, and burned out.[1] In addition, their long hours and consecutive shifts can add to the likelihood of burnout. In one study, 30% to 50% of physicians surveyed indicated that they would not go into medical school if they were to begin their career again, and they would encourage their children to pursue a different path.[6]

Nurses can also be prone to burnout. In fact, 40% of hospital nurses have burnout levels that exceed the norms for health care workers.[7] Caring for patients who often cannot effectively communicate their gratitude can put a strain on a nurse. In addition, staffing shortages, mandatory overtime, and extended shifts can exacerbate the likelihood of burnout. Nurses working in areas where patients are unlikely to recover from their illnesses or whose illnesses require intense treatment, such as within the intensive care unit, can be particularly prone to burnout. Nurses who provide care to children with incurable diseases might also be more likely than others to experience burnout.

In addition to physicians and nurses, social workers, emergency service personnel, and mental health professionals can suffer from burnout as the day-to-day demands of these jobs can take a toll on even the most optimistic professionals.

More Information: Compassion Fatigue

A specific type of burnout that is often experienced by health care workers is called *compassion fatigue*. This term refers to a gradual lessening of compassion over time. It results from the taxing nature of showing compassion for someone whose suffering is continuous and unresolvable. One might still care for the person out of a sense of duty, obligation, or necessity; however, the natural human desire to help the ailing person is no longer there.[8]

Specifically within the health care arena, those individuals who are primary care providers for patients with terminal illnesses are at increased risk of developing compassion fatigue. For example, nurses on an oncology ward, staff members caring for Alzheimer's patients, and other staff caring for people with long-term, unresolving illnesses can suffer from this phenomenon.[8] If not addressed, compassion fatigue can lead to abusive behavior by the caregiver to care recipients and can also lead to depression, stress, and trauma.

The Signs of Burnout

There are many signs of burnout, and they tend to be more mental than physical. In fact, many of the indications of health care worker burnout can be seen in the quality of care an individual provides to patients. Following are a few of the signs of which to be aware:

- Powerlessness and hopelessness
- Emotional exhaustion
- Detachment and isolation
- Irritability and frustration
- A feeling of being trapped
- Failure
- Despair
- Cynicism
- Apathy[9]
- Lack of personal accomplishment
- Depersonalization

People who are becoming burned out might frequently snap at people or make snide remarks. They might experience depression or antisocial behavior. In some severe cases, worker burnout can lead to destructive behavior, such as chronic alcohol issues, drug problems, or suicide.

More Information: Blaming the Employee

Often, when an individual is burned out, he or she might feel it is his or her fault. In some cases, the employer also chooses to examine the personal characteristics of the employee, citing character flaws or personality traits as the main contributors to burnout. However, it is thought that the social environment and organizational structure in the work environment are more relevant to burnout than are personal characteristics.[10]

How Does Burnout Happen?

Many factors can cause burnout, including prolonged stress with little abatement, role ambiguity in a job, inadequate training or orientation to a job, lack of social support, long work hours, repetitive night duty, perpetually rotating shift work, continuous lack of sleep, and economic uncertainty. Things like increased overtime—particularly when it is required and not optional—and lengthy shift work can also lead to burnout. Burnout does not come on suddenly, and an individual might not even be aware that he or she is experiencing burnout.

Measuring Burnout

To ensure the most productive staff and the highest-quality care, organizations should determine whether staff members are experiencing burnout. There are a variety of ways to do this, including conducting surveys, engaging in walk-arounds to ask staff about burnout, and conducting focus groups. Organizations can also collect from employee records information that could signal potential burnout. Such information might include excessive absenteeism, tardiness, inordinate use of sick leave, or other evidence of workplace avoidance.[1]

The most studied tool for measuring burnout is the Maslach Burnout Inventory (MBI).[11] This tool is designed to measure an "enduring state of experienced burnout" and patterns of burnout among groups of workers.[11] The MBI assesses three components of burnout:

1. **Emotional exhaustion:** This component addresses the feelings of being emotionally overextended and exhausted by one's work.
2. **Depersonalization:** This component addresses the level of unfeeling or impersonal response toward recipients of care, treatment, and services.
3. **Reduced personal accomplishment:** This component assesses feelings of competence and successful achievement with one's work.

The survey contains 22 items that are written in the form of statements about personal feelings or attitudes. For example, some of the statements include "I feel burned out from my work" and "I don't really care what happens to some recipients." The items are answered in terms of the frequency in which the respondent experiences these feelings, ranging from 0, which means "never," to 6, meaning "every day," The MBI takes approximately 10 to 15 minutes to fill out and is self-administered.[11]

Consequences of Burnout

Burnout can have several negative consequences. It can lead to degraded performance, decreased efficiency, increased absenteeism, and increased job turnover. On a personal level, burnout can lead to physical and behavioral changes, including depression, exhaustion, weight loss or gain, muscle pain, headaches, respiratory illnesses, gastrointestinal disorders, hypertension, and insomnia.[1] In serious cases, burnout sometimes leads to substance and chemical abuse as well as marital and family problems.

Burnout can become a patient safety issue, as caregivers who are burned out might not be paying as close attention to their patients as they should, might not get to know their patients as well as they should, and can have a hard time focusing on the task at hand. They might overlook issues, miss critical windows of opportunity, and fail to go the extra mile to care for their patients. A correlation between burned-out health care workers and low patient satisfaction has also been shown.[10]

The Differences Between Stress and Burnout

Burnout might be a result of unrelenting stress but it isn't the same as stress (*see* Table 4-1, on page 91). Stress, by and large, involves too much of something, such as too much pressure, too many demands, too many deadlines, too many competing priorities, or too much physical exertion. However, stressed people can still imagine that if they can just get everything under control, they'll feel better.[9]

Burnout, on the other hand, deals with the concept of not enough. Being burned out means feeling empty, devoid of motivation, and beyond caring. People

Table 4-1.
Characteristics of Stress Versus Burnout

Stress	Burnout
– Characterized by over-engagement	– Characterized by disengagement
– Emotions are over-reactive	– Emotions are blunted
– Produces urgency and hyperactivity	– Produces helplessness and hopelessness
– Loss of energy	– Loss of motivation, ideals, and hope
– Leads to anxiety disorders	– Leads to detachment and depression
– Primary damage is physical	– Primary damage is emotional
– Might kill you prematurely	– Might make life seem not worth living

Source: Adapted from Croucher R.: *Stress and Burnout in Ministry*. http://www.churchlink.com.au/churchlink/forum/r_croucher/stress_burnout.html (accessed Dec. 10, 2007).

experiencing burnout often don't see any hope of positive change in their situations. If excessive stress is like drowning in responsibilities, burnout is like being all dried up.[9]

Strategies to Prevent Worker Burnout

As with addressing worker fatigue and sleep deprivation, there is no one guaranteed solution to preventing and addressing burnout. However, there are some common methods of attacking the problem that could prove useful when implemented in an environment that supports teamwork and communication. Some common ways to help combat burnout include the following:

- **Addressing compensation issues:** This might involve ensuring fair and appropriate compensation for all staff. Compensation can reflect the value an organization places on its workers. Although most health care workers do not choose to pursue the profession because of the money, fair compensation can help them maintain a positive outlook toward work.
- **Providing comprehensive benefits:** Almost more important than the compensation are the benefits an organization provides to its employees. These can show how much the organization cares for its employees on a personal level, as benefits deal with employees' personal lives. Benefits do not just include health insurance and a 401(k) plan but may also include flexible schedules, tuition reimbursement, flexible spending accounts, gym memberships, child-care options, and so forth.
- **Increasing an individual's control over his or her job:** This could include fostering an environment where staff members help design schedules, are

involved in determining and adjusting job responsibilities, and see direct lines of growth and improvement. To truly involve individuals in their jobs, organizations should commit to reexamining job descriptions and responsibilities regularly.

- **Providing access to employee assistance programs (EAPs):** An EAP is a counseling service for employees (and, often, their eligible dependents) who might be experiencing personal or workplace problems. Typically, an EAP is available around the clock. An EAP can address a wide range of problems, including, but not limited to, the following:
    - Emotional problems
    - Family issues
    - Marital conflicts
    - Stress-related issues
    - Financial problems
    - Substance abuse issues
    - Legal problems
    - Workplace struggles
    - Elder-care issues

    Sometimes an EAP might provide consultation or referral services as well.

Ensuring Appropriate Staffing

Insufficient staffing is a big contributor to burnout in health care workers. One study showed that increased emotional exhaustion and job dissatisfaction in nurses were strongly and significantly associated with patient-to-nurse ratios.[7]

Current staffing shortages have pushed health care providers to do more with fewer resources, and staff members are under intense pressure to assess and respond to patients' needs quickly. Individuals working in an environment where they must work longer, harder, and faster in order to meet the demands of the department can lead to exhaustion, fatigue, stress, and, ultimately, burnout.

In some cases, staff members who are not suitably qualified to handle certain situations, such as surgery, are being asked to work in these areas because of staffing shortages. A person being put in a work environment for which he or she is not qualified can cause undue amounts of prolonged stress and thus lead to burnout.

Health care leaders must develop and implement effective strategies for addressing staffing issues to reduce the likelihood of worker burnout. These could include strategies for hiring, retaining, and scheduling staff. Although there are many ways to address staffing within an organization, organizations might want to consider the following suggestions when dealing with staffing issues.

Hire the right people for the job. Selecting the right person for a particular position can help improve performance for the health care team, not to mention morale. Conversely, hiring the wrong person can create performance deficits and staff dissatisfaction.[12] When considering a hiring strategy, organizations should try to structure the interview process to yield not only qualified candidates but ones who will fit the corporate culture and meet the performance expectations and competency requirements of the job. This can be done by tailoring interview questions to specifically assess the likelihood of superior job performance. Such questions could include direct questions about job skills, questions designed to reveal underlying aspects of the candidate's attitude and approach to his or her job, and questions that can cause the candidate to reveal his or her own strengths and weaknesses.[12] To create these questions, an organization should consider the goals of the position, any job barriers that exist that would prevent an individual from reaching the goals, and any competency requirements necessary to reach the goals. When determining goals for a position, an organization should be as specific as possible. When determining job barriers, an organization should consider both the individual's barriers to success and any organizational barriers to success.[12] In addition to asking the right questions, an organization should ensure that it provides the candidate with all the information to make an informed choice about the organization. For example, information should be given to the candidate about the organization's culture, performance expectations, emphasis on performance improvement, and perspective on patient involvement. An informed applicant can make a better decision about whether he or she is a good fit for the organization.

Foster an environment of retention. The sense of connectedness fostered through teamwork and collegial communication is a powerful staff retention tool. Organizations best able to recruit and retain staff offer an environment characterized by mutual respect and high-quality communication among nurses, physicians, and other staff.

Cross-train staff for multifunctionality. Cross-training can help ensure that appropriately qualified and competent staff members are available to relieve fatigued workers, overburdened workers, or individuals who opt for a scheduled nap. Organizations that successfully cross-train assign staff members to a primary department but cross-train them to work competently and effectively in other areas. For example, medical/surgical nurses can be cross-trained to assist in the emergency room, postanesthesia care units, and same-day surgery centers. When training, it is important to consider how a staff member will be cross-trained to function in the different patient care teams and ensure that he or she receives proper teamwork and communication training.

Consider whether certain tasks can be delegated responsibly and appropriately, and if they can, do so. To ease the load on the most stressed staff members—for example, surgical registered nurses—organizations should consider allowing staff with the appropriate skill mix to work under the direction of a registered nurse and perform some of the most routine care tasks. Appropriate delegation with supervision can help eliminate unachievable workloads.

Pay attention to work schedules. The majority of employees have identified the need for balance between personal and work lives as one of the most important determinants of job satisfaction.[13] Flexible work schedules represent a major job benefit for many employees. Organizations might want to consider offering the option of flexible work schedules for their employees. These could include schedules allowing 7 days on full time and 7 days off; 10-hour shifts 4 days a week; or 12-hour shifts 3 days a week. When designing flexible work schedules, organizations should make sure that they allow health care workers to catch up on sleep between shifts and provide the opportunity to get adequate rest.

Commit resources to hire more staff. Although many organizations are feeling the pinch of the staffing shortage, organizations would be wise to commit resources to address staffing deficits, when possible. Oftentimes, if resources are spent wisely, an organization can recoup any costs for additional staff through increased productivity, worker retention, and a reduction in expensive errors. For example, a hospital that invests in a nocturnist position can often recoup that investment through reduced errors and increased patient throughput.

Helping Workers Manage Stress

As previously mentioned, too much stress or stress that does not abate is a primary cause of worker burnout. One way to prevent worker burnout is to provide workers access to tools to combat stress. Such tools might include the following.

Coping strategies. Coping strategies cover a wide range of activities that individuals can do to manage stress. Although these activities do not necessarily eliminate stress, they do help people cope, manage, and work through stress. The following are some coping strategies:

- Listening to music
- Writing in a journal
- Talking with a friend
- Exercising
- Sleeping

- Meditating or praying
- Drinking herbal tea

Relaxation techniques. An individual can relax his or her mind and body in a number of ways. Some specific relaxation techniques from which health care workers can benefit include yoga, tai chi, focused mediation, and massage.

Mental imagery techniques. Mental imagery techniques allow individuals to focus on a problem and project how they will address, minimize, or eliminate the problem. Such techniques involve seeing the positive outcomes of stressful situations and imagining how to navigate those situations to achieve the envisioned outcomes.

Support groups. Oftentimes, people can relieve stress by talking with others who are experiencing similar situations or who have experienced and progressed through specific situations. Support groups offer an opportunity for people with like issues to come together and garner support and encouragement from each other. Usually support groups center around a particular topic, such as alcoholism, tragic loss, parenting, or a particular health issue, such as cancer or AIDS.

Counseling services. Many people find help from the counseling of a professional. Health care organizations are in a good position to provide such professional services through psychologists, social workers, clergy, and so forth.

One of the best ways to provide access to these tools is through education and training. Organizations might wish to provide stress management training within their facilities or provide access to such training at remote locations. Some good sources for stress management information can be found in Sidebar 4-1 on page 96. Health care organizations might also wish to support the creation of support groups or provide access to counseling services.

Recognizing and Rewarding Accomplishments

An important step in preventing burnout is to recognize and reward individuals for their hard work, accomplishments, and achievements. Staff members work best in an environment that makes them feel valued—where they get a "thank you" for a job well done.

Rewarding and recognizing good performance can have the following effects:

- Increase staff commitment to an organization's or an initiative's goals
- Attract and retain outstanding staff
- Foster a positive, constructive, and productive work environment
- Provide for ongoing learning

Sidebar 4-1. Sources for Stress Management Information

Centers for Disease Control and Prevention
http://www.cdc.gov

American Institute of Stress
http://www.stress.org

Mayo Clinic's Stress Center
http://www.mayoclinic.com/health/stress/SR99999

VA National Center for Patient Safety http://www.va.gov/ncps/

- Promote collaboration
- Enhance staff satisfaction

Rewards for good performance can take a variety of forms, including the following:

- A simple "thank you"
- Informal acknowledgements either face-to-face or via e-mail
- Letters of appreciation from a more senior manager
- Public recognition in front of peers, such as at staff meetings, group luncheons, or organizationwide meetings
- Posted lists or testimonials about good performers in break rooms, company newsletters, group e-mails, and so forth
- Small gifts, such as mugs, t-shirts, gift certificates to restaurants, or vouchers for the cafeteria
- Publicity, such as mentions in company newsletters and on intranet sites
- More frequent assignment to duties the staff member likes
- Opportunities for advanced training
- Monetary bonuses

The best source of information about which staff members are performing well or achieving great things is peer reports and nominations. These can be obtained through a variety of methods, including discussions with nurse managers, recommendation forms, e-mail solicitations, and so forth.

When an organization meets its goals regarding a particular initiative—especially if staff members have worked long hours and sacrificed their personal time to meet an initiative's goals—it is a significant milestone that warrants celebration. A celebration can help underscore the importance of an initiative and encourage staff to "keep up the good work." Celebrations convey that leadership is pleased with the efforts of staff and is rewarding the improved behavior.

Organization leaders shouldn't do a half-hearted job planning a celebration. Budget restraints might determine what kind of celebration is held, but choices can include an on-site gathering or a group dinner at a nearby restaurant. The type of celebration will depend on the staff involved with the initiative. More important than budget is that the celebration reflect something the participants enjoy. Some things to consider when planning a celebration include the following:

- How many people should be included in the celebration?
- What will everyone enjoy?
- What will be relaxing?
- What will be different enough from the usual socializing to mark this as a special occasion?

For example, an organization that uses a sports theme in a performance improvement initiative might want to consider taking staff members to a baseball game when the initiative is successfully implemented.

Nothing augments praise like amplification. Initiative leaders should send an e-mail or post a memo to announce the celebration. Alert the organization's senior managers about the celebration and invite them to attend. Even if they don't come, staff members will appreciate the fact that their success was communicated to upper management.

Organization leaders should listen carefully during celebrations. Leadership can learn a great deal by taking the opportunity to observe staff in this more casual environment. This kind of relaxed event might produce more candid conversation than a formal project meeting. If staff members are expressing their concerns or problems with a project, an initiative, or a process, pay close attention.[14] These concerns and worries can provide suggestions for the next time.

Ensuring Appropriate Orientation and Training

Burnout can occur when an individual is not adequately prepared for the role he or she plays in the organization. This can lead to job ambiguity, fear of failure, a sense of hopelessness and confusion, and ultimately burnout. Effective orientation and training can help prevent worker burnout because they help introduce individuals to an organization and their jobs, ensure that they have the necessary knowledge and skills to competently perform their jobs, keep them abreast of new developments in their fields, and improve in areas where their competence is deficient. Good orientation and training programs can help motivate employees, reduce turnover, increase productivity, improve morale, decrease the likelihood of burnout, and facilitate systemwide learning.[15]

All individuals working in or for a hospital must receive orientation and training, including licensed independent practitioners, direct care and non–direct care staff, contract staff, and students. Orientation and training programs should not be limited to full-time staff members but should also include volunteers, part-time workers, and contract employees as well.

The orientation and training process can be broken down into several different components:

- Orientation for new hires
- Orientation for a new role or job
- Training to maintain competence

Orientation for new hires. The Joint Commission requires hospitals to have an orientation process that provides each individual who works for the hospital with initial job training and information and that assesses the individual's ability to fulfill specified responsibilities. This orientation process familiarizes new staff members with their jobs and the work environment before they begin patient care or other activities. It focuses on the individual's role in the organization and the importance of his or her function.

A hospital should have well-defined policies and procedures outlining the type of orientation required for individuals working for the organization. Orientation is a two- or three-stage process that covers general hospitalwide job competencies and specific departmental and position competencies. It offers the opportunity for individuals to understand what is expected of them as well as what they can expect from the organization.

Topics covered in each stage of orientation should be outlined in the hospital's overall competence assessment plan or policies. Department- and job-specific orientations should not duplicate what is covered in the general orientation but should complement and supplement it with more specific material related to the individual's specific role.

General orientation. General hospitalwide orientation provides information that is critical to all individuals, wherever they work in the organization, and should introduce an employee to the structure, culture, and standards of an organization. General orientation usually includes, but is not limited to, the following topics:

- Hospital mission, vision, and values
- The hospital's performance improvement program
- Safety and emergency management policies and procedures
- Work environment and environment of care issues
- Infection control policies and procedures
- Benefits and personnel policies
- Cultural competence training
- Communication, interpersonal skills, and team training

Department-specific orientation. Department-specific orientation drills down from general orientation to include topics that relate more specifically to particular

More Information: Orientation for New Graduates

When an individual is not only new to an organization but new to a profession, a comprehensive orientation process is critical. Organizations might want to consider adding a component to new graduates' orientation process and have each new graduate work with a mentor, coach, or preceptor for a defined period of time. A preceptor program pairs a more experienced staff person or practitioner with a new employee or practitioner. This method has been shown to be effective in orienting new staff to an organization, and it can help to increase staff satisfaction and retention as well. The experienced staff person serves as a facilitator and resource person for orienting the new staff person to the organization.[16]

Preceptors should be experienced in the organization, be willing to act as preceptors, and have some additional training on how to train new employees. It is important when pairing a preceptor with a new employee to match the preceptor's teaching style to the learning style of the new employee. At the conclusion of the preceptor relationship, the preceptor would be in a position to assess the individual's competence and recommend him or her for independent practice.

Another option for supplementing a new graduate's orientation program is an internship period. During such a period, the graduate would rotate through a variety of areas within the organization to get a better picture of how the organization functions and his or her role in it.

departments. Department-specific orientation generally includes topics such as the following:

- Departmental policies and procedures
- Patient safety issues, policies, and procedures
- Description of the key functions and tasks performed in the department or unit
- Equipment and skills needed for the tasks performed in the department or unit
- Job-specific safety issues
- The individual's role in the department

Job-specific orientation. Job-specific orientation drills down even further from department-specific orientation and addresses the issues with which an individual must be familiar to perform his or her job. Depending on the organization and the position, some hospitals choose to combine the department-specific and job-specific orientations. Some job-specific orientation topics include the following:

- Elements of the individual's job description
- Specific performance expectations and competencies

- Skills and equipment specific to the position that will be validated by a manager or supervisor

All individuals must be assessed after completing the orientation process. According to Joint Commission standards, a hospital's orientation process must include an evaluation of an individual's ability to perform the job for which he or she has been hired. Assessment of the individual's competence to perform specific assigned duties during the orientation process establishes a baseline from which further competence assessment and training can be done.

At the end of the orientation process, an individual must be competent to perform the skills specified in his or her job description. If an individual is found not competent during the post-orientation assessment, further training is required. This training could take many forms, including the use of a proctor or mentor, further training programs, audiovisual instruction materials, and so forth.

Orientation for a New Role or Position

An orientation is not just reserved for new employees to an organization. If an individual is beginning a new job or role in the organization, he or she should be oriented to that role. Like new-hire orientation, this orientation should include the specific performance expectations and competencies of the new role, as well as a discussion of any new skills or equipment necessary to competently perform the job. At the completion of this orientation process, the individual's competency should be tested before he or she is allowed to perform his or her job independently.

Training to Maintain Competence

The education of individuals does not stop with the orientation process. An organization must also have a training process that fosters staff development and continued learning. Skill deficiencies are also addressed in training programs.

Training needs arise every day in a hospital, such as when new equipment or medications are introduced, when new policies are created, when new developments in the field arise, and when the hospital's data collection indicates a need for training. In addition, organizations should support practitioners' and staff members' continuing education goals and requirements. This might include providing tuition reimbursement, days off for off-site education programs, and so forth.

Assessing the Success of an Orientation and Training Program

Orientation and training is a performance improvement activity, and as with other performance improvement activity, organizations should periodically assess its effectiveness. This can be done through a variety of methods, including the following:

More Information: Instructional Methods for Orientation and Training

Orientation and training should be interactive, engaging, and thought provoking. Whether an organization's program fits this description is dependent in part on the types of methods used for instruction. Instructional or educational methods used during orientation and training should be varied based on the individuals receiving the education. Physicians, for example, might respond best to self-instruction, online courses, teleconferences, or written information, as the time they have available for in-services and on-site training sessions might be limited. Nurses who are being trained to perform a specific skill might respond best to one-on-one instruction, return demonstration, or simulation efforts.

Instructional methods should also vary depending on the topic being covered. The following are possible educational methods:

- Lectures or classes
- Audiovisual programs
- Written materials
- Group discussions and other interactive activities
- One-on-one instruction
- Demonstration and return demonstration
- Simulation and role-playing
- Self-instruction modules
- Online instruction

When determining what methods to use for education, it is important to keep in mind that the use of multiple learning methods can increase the likelihood that skills will be acquired and retained. Creativity is often needed to design programs that are effective from both education and cost perspectives.

Because everyone learns differently, it is helpful to identify individuals' preferred or best ways of learning during the orientation process. For example, some people retain more information if they hear material rather than having it presented in written form. Others can more readily grasp a technique by performing it themselves under the guidance of an instructor than by watching someone else do it. Active learning almost always leads to better retention than lecturing alone. Many hospitals therefore hold skills days or equipment days during which employees can learn new skills or new technology and can review existing procedures in an informal atmosphere.

Orientation and training programs should be tailored to the audience being trained.

(continued)

More Information: Instructional Methods for Orientation and Training (continued)

For example, volunteers might not necessarily have the clinical background to fully understand the importance of an issue such as infection control. In the instance of training a volunteer on infection control issues, training materials should focus on ways to reduce the spread of infection, such as appropriate hand washing techniques.

Orientation and training programs should also consider the unique needs of the staff receiving the training. For example, non-English-speaking staff might require an interpreter at the time of orientation.

- Staff surveys or focus groups
- Pre- and posttests
- Return demonstration activities

For example, if an organization's orientation and training programs consistently receive low satisfaction scores from staff members, this might indicate the need to tweak the program. Similarly, after looking at aggregate scores for all individuals taking a particular course, an organization can determine whether the program is effective as a whole. An aggregate increase in score can indicate a successful program, whereas an aggregate decrease or no change in score can signify a program that needs improvement.

Creating a Burnout-Reducing Environment

Another strategy that can help prevent burnout is establishing a positive, comfortable, and pleasing environment in which to work. People are sensitive to their surroundings, and being surrounded by a pleasing atmosphere can make a difference in their performance, attitude, stress level, and outlook. Noisy, stressful, cheerless work environments contribute to staff fatigue, stress, burnout, and poor performance. These environmental factors are pushing up nurse turnover rates. The following are some ways organizations can alter the environment to help reduce staff stress and prevent burnout.

Using nature to enhance the environment. Plants, fountains, waterfalls, gardens, and natural views can reduce staff and patient stress, improve morale, and lead to positive clinical outcomes. Access to nature can diminish negative emotions, such as fear and anger, and increase positive feelings. Viewing nature or paintings of nature can result in physiological changes, including reduced blood pressure and heart activity. On the other hand, studies suggest that looking at built scenes that lack nature, such as rooms, buildings, and parking lots, can increase stress.[12] When considering the environment, organizations should try to include skylights, windows, atriums, and other design elements throughout the building to provide patient and staff access to natural light and nature.

Ensuring good air quality. The quality of air in an environment not only can prevent the spread of infection and disease but can also improve mood, outlook, and attitude. Organizations should consider the most effective ways to keep the air "clean" in order to improve patient outcomes and staff productivity. Clean air can also help reduce absenteeism and improve worker safety. To achieve good air quality, an organization should make sure it has the proper ventilation and air filtration.

Letting in the light. Staff should have adequate light in order to clearly see medication labels, charts, computer keyboards, and so forth. This light should be directed so that staff can use it without waking or disturbing patients. Some organizations prefer to use indirect artificial lighting versus natural lighting, as it still provides the benefits of light while creating a more home-like ambiance.

Using art to create peace. Like nature, artwork can help reduce stress and promote positive feelings. However, the impact of art is related to the type of art used. Artwork that depicts nature scenes, such as flowers, seascapes, and mountains, can promote positive feelings and reduce stress. On the other hand, abstract art can sometimes increase stress.

Providing access to music. Soft music can help reduce stress and increase positive feelings in a health care environment. Grand pianos playing in lobbies and relaxing music in patient care areas can help provide a home-like environment and improve patient well-being and staff outlook.

Use home-like designs. Many health care facilities today are cold, impersonal spaces that seem to communicate a lack of caring. By incorporating soft colors on the walls, comfortable furniture, indirect lighting, artwork, and so forth, organizations can communicate that the health care facility is a healing and supportive environment where staff members care for patients and value their well-being.

Moving toward a decentralized design. Many health care facilities have a central nurses' station on each unit where charts, orders, medications, and supplies are stored. Nurses in these facilities spend significant time walking up and down hallways to gather what they need for patient care. A recent study by Ann Hendrich and her colleagues used video cameras to track how nurses spend their days. They found that, on average, nurses spent only about 30 to 40 minutes of their shifts actually giving care at the bedside because of the time spent searching for and gathering supplies.[18] In addition to pulling nurses away from patient care, crowded, noisy workstations add to staff stress, reduce effective communication, and can lead to medical errors. Decentralized floor plans allow nurses to work closer to patients, thus reducing the need to hunt for supplies. Evidence shows that these floor plans can reduce staff stress, increase satisfaction, and allow nurses to respond more quickly to patient needs.[18]

Reducing unnecessary noise. Hospital noise comes from loud equipment, multiple voices speaking at once, overhead paging systems, and so forth. At the same time, environmental surfaces, such as floors, walls, and ceilings, are typically not sound absorbing—and can, in fact, amplify noise.[19] Prolonged exposure to environmental noise can increase stress and agitation and also reduce concentration and limit communication. To help improve noise levels, organizations should consider the following actions:

- Install sound-absorbing ceiling tiles or wall panels
- Carpet hallways to reduce the noise of moving equipment
- Decentralize nursing stations, where nurses, phyicians, and other health care staff tend to congregate and talk
- Build single-patient rooms
- Mask noxious sounds with pleasant sounds, such as classical music or nature sounds
- Train staff to be aware of noise levels and teach them how to reduce them, such as by speaking more softly and turning off cell phones
- Eliminate overhead paging systems[20]

Providing mobile charting. An organization can increase staff efficiency and reduce fatigue by using mobile charting. Mobile charting stations can be moved about a unit and docked at "charting islands." This allows quick access to patient information and flexibility of patient care.[21]

Using cushioned flooring materials. Because nurses spend the majority of their day on their feet, the type of flooring material used in a health care facility can affect the comfort, health, and safety of staff. Cushioned materials, such as carpet or sheet vinyl with a padded backing, can dramatically improve staff performance and satisfaction.

More Information: Sources for Orientation and Training Information

In addition to considering the format of educational materials, organizations should also consider the content of those materials. The sources for orientation and training content can vary depending on the topic being covered. Some sources include the following:

- Internal sources, such as the human resources department and organization leadership
- Government sources, such as the Centers for Disease Control and Prevention (CDC), Health Resources and Services Administration (HRSA), Centers for Medicare & Medicaid Services (CMS), U.S. Department of Health and Human Services (HHS) Office of Minority Health, and Veterans Health Administration (VHA)
- Professional associations, such as the American Nursing Association (ANA), American Medical Association (AMA), American College of Surgeons (ACS), Association of periOperative Registered Nurses (AORN), American Pharmacists Association (AphA), and American College of Healthcare Executives (ACHE)
- Not-for-profit organizations, such as the Institute for Healthcare Improvement, the Institute for Safe Medication Practices, and the National Patient Safety Foundation
- Other hospitals and health care organizations

Designing ergonomic nurses' stations. Shelves that are too high, outlets that are too low, and computer workstations that stress the hands and wrists can all lead to worker injuries, absenteeism, burnout, and an unsafe work environment. Organizations that design the environment to limit staff reaching, bending, twisting, and stretching can improve staff safety, health, and satisfaction.

Grouping similar patient care areas together. Staff spend a lot of time during the day walking between different patient care areas. For example, one patient might need to have an x-ray and a CT scan. If the areas that house these two procedures are not located near each other, a staff member might spend time and energy walking from department to department. Layouts that group like patient care areas together, such as imaging services, can limit the amount of walking necessary.

Providing respite areas. Respite areas are places staff and patients can go to relax, meditate, pray, and so forth. Areas such as gardens, music rooms, and chapels can provide a place for staff to rejuvenate and recharge before returning to work.

Organizations have a responsibility to address staff needs in the environment, not only because of the safety implications of not addressing staff needs but because it is the right thing to do. Consider the words of one expert: "Think of the impact on the staff of cramped quarters, inadequate lighting and personal storage space, long walks between patient rooms, and distraction-prone work spaces. How can you expect employees to 'go above and beyond' with patients and their families when you haven't provided work environments conducive to the employees' own physical and psychological health?"[23]

Conclusion

Worker burnout can be a potentially serious issue for both individuals and organizations. However, addressing burnout and putting in place strategies to prevent burnout does not have to be complex. Although there is no one solution, organizations can implement a variety of strategies that can reduce stress, improve attitude, reduce absenteeism, prevent burnout, and ultimately improve performance.

References

1. Felton J.S.: Burnout as a clinical entity: Its importance in health care workers. *Occup Med* (*Lond*) 48:237–250, 1998.

2. *Burnout.* http://en.wikipedia.org/wiki/Burnout (accessed Dec. 10, 2007).

3. Penson R., et al.: Burnout: Caring for the caregivers. *Oncologist* 5:425–434, 2000.

4. Maslach C.: Burned-out. *Human Behavior* 4:16–22, 1976.

5. Cordes, C., Dougherty, T.: A review and integration of research on job burnout. *Academy of Management Review* 18:621–656, 1993.

6. Lambert C.: Dissatisfied doctors. *Harvard Magazine* 96:19–20, 1993.

7. Aiken L., et al.: Hospital nurse staffing and patient mortality, nurse burnout, and job satisfaction. *JAMA* 288:1987–1993, Oct. 2002.

8. *Compassion Fatigue.* http://en.wikipedia.org/wiki/Compassion_fatigue (accessed Dec. 10, 2007).

9. *Preventing Burnout: Signs, Symptoms, and Strategies to Avoid It.* http://www.helpguide.org/mental/burnout_signs_symptoms.htm (accessed Dec. 7, 2007.)

10. Medland J.: Fostering psychosocial wellness in oncology nurses: Addressing burnout and social support in the workplace. Oncol Nurs Forum 31:47–54, 2004.

11. Maslach C., et al: *Maslach Burnout Inventory, Third Ed.* Consulting Psychologists Press, Mountain View California.

12. Nierenberg R.: The use of a strategic interviewing technique to select the nurse manager. *J Nurs Adm* 33:500–505, 2003.

13. Izzo J.B., Withers P.: Winning employee-retention strategies for today's healthcare organizations. Healthc Financ Manage, pp 52–57, Jun. 2002.

14. Robinson S.: *How to Celebrate Team Success*, Nov.12, 2002. http://builder.com.com/5100-6315-1049991.html (accessed Feb. 2, 2005).

15. Ragsdale M., Mueller J.: Plan, do, study, act model to improve an orientation program. *J Nurs Care Qual* 30:268–272, 2005.

16. Harper J.: Preceptors' perceptions of a competency based orientation. *J Nurses Staff Dev* 18(4):198–202, 2002.

17. Ulrich R., et al.: *The Role of the Physical Environment in the Hospital of the 21st Century: A Once-in-a-Lifetime Opportunity.* http://www.healthdesign.org/research/reports/physical_environ.php (accessed Dec. 10, 2007).

18. McCarthy M.: Healthy design. *Lancet* 364:405–406, Jul. 31, 2004.

19. Center for Health Design releases findings on how design can improve the standard of care in health-care facilities. *AIArchitect*, Feb. 21, 2005. http://www.aia.org/aiarchitect/thisweek05/tw0218/0218bp_pebble.htm (accessed Dec. 10, 2007).

20. Mazer S.: Stop: Reduce errors by creating a quieter hospital environment. *Patient Safety & Quality Healthcare* pp. 36–39, Mar.–Apr. 2005.

21. Leighty J.: Healing by design. *NurseWeek*, Apr. 23, 2003. http://www.nurseweek.com/news/features/03-04/unitfuture.asp (accessed Dec. 10 2005).

22. Hobstetter D.: In the Fray: Seeing the light about daylight. *Wall Street Journal*, Oct. 19, 2004.

23. Center for Health Design.: Design for success: Efficiency and effectiveness through facility design. Healthc Financ Manage, pp. DE1–DE13, Nov. 2003.

APPENDIX ONE

Suggested Readings

Resources on Fatigue and Sleep Deprivation

- Arora V.: Improving the sleep hygiene of medical interns. *Arch Intern Med* 167:1738–1744, Sep. 10, 2007.

- Arora V., et al.: The effects of on-duty napping on intern sleep time and fatigue. *Ann Intern Med* 144:792–798, 2006.

- Barger L.K., et al.: Extended work shifts and the risk of motor vehicle crashes among interns. *N Engl J Med* 13:125–134, Jan. 13, 2005.

- Beyea S.: Too tired to work safely. *AORN J* 80:559–560, Sep. 2004.

- Blachowicz E., Letizia M.: The challenges of shift work. *Medsurg Nurs* 15:274–280, Oct. 2006.

- Caruso C., Condon M.: Night shifts and fatigue: Coping skills for the working nurse. *Am J Nurs* 106:88, Aug. 2006.

- Dawson D., et al.: Fatigue, alcohol, and performance impairment. *Nature* 388:235, Jul. 17, 1997.

- Eastridge B.J., et al.: Effects of sleep deprivation on the performance of simulated laparoscopic surgical skill. *Am J Surg* 186:169–174, Aug. 2003.

- Fatigue in healthcare workers. *Healthcare Risk Control. Risk Analysis Employment Issues* 14 (Suppl. A), Jan. 2006.

- Fatigue in the workplace is common and costly. *Medical News Today*, Jan. 15, 2007. http://www.medicalnewstoday.com/medicalnews.php?newsid=60732 (accessed Dec. 1, 2007).
- Gaba D.M., Howard S.K.: Patient safety: Fatigue among clinicians and the safety of patients. *N Engl J Med* 17:129–155, Oct. 17, 2002.
- Gurchiek K.: Study finds eye-opening cost associated with fatigued workers. *HR News*, Jan. 30, 2007.
- Howard S.K., et al.: Fatigue in anesthesia: Implications and strategies for patient and provider safety. *Anesthesiology* 97:1281–1294, 2002.
- Howard S., et al.: The risks and implications of excessive daytime sleepiness in resident physicians. *Acad Med* 77:1019–1025, Oct. 2002.
- Lockley S., et al.: Effects of health care provider work hours and sleep deprivation on safety and performance. *Jt Comm J Qual Patient Saf* 33:7–18, Nov. 2007.
- Muecke S.: Effects of rotating night shifts: A literature review. *J Adv Nurs* 30:433–439, 2005.
- Nevarez M., Howard S.: Fatigue in anesthesia: The impact on patient and provider safety: Update on work-hour limitations. *Advances in Anesthesia* 21:85–107, 2006.
- Olson L., Ambrogetti A.: Working harder—Working dangerously? Fatigue and performance in hospitals. *Med J Aust* 168:614–616, 1998.
- Papp K., et al.: The effects of sleep loss and fatigue on resident-physicians: A multi-institutional, mixed-method study. *Acad Med* 79: 394–406, May 2004.
- Poissonnet C.M., Veron M.: Health effects of work schedules in healthcare professions. *J Clin Nurs* 9:13–23, Jan. 2000.
- Rogers A.E., et al.: The working hours of hospital staff nurses and patient safety. *Health Aff (Millwood)* 23:202–212, Jul.–Aug. 2004.
- Rosekind M.: Managing work schedules: An alertness and safety perspective.

In Kryger M., Roth T., Dement W. (eds.): *Principles and Practice of Sleep Medicine.* Philadelphia: Elsevier Science, 2005, pp. 680–690.

- Rosekind M.: Managing fatigue 24/7 in health care: Opportunities to improve safety. *Anesthesia Patient Safety Foundation Newsletter* vol. 20, Spring 2005. http://www.apsf.org/resource_center/newsletter/2005/spring/06managing.htm. (accessed Dec. 1, 2007).

- Rosekind M.R., et al.: Alertness management: Strategic naps in operational settings. *J Sleep Res* 3:62–66, 1995.

- Scott L., Hwang W., Rogers A.: The impact of multiple care giving roles on fatigue, stress, and work performance among hospital staff nurses. *J Nurs Adm* 36:86–95, Feb. 2006.

- National Sleep Foundation: *2002 "Sleep in America" Poll,* Mar. 2002. http://www.kintera.org/atf/cf/%7BF6BF2668-A1B4-4FE8-8D1A-A5D39340D9CB%7D/2002SleepInAmericaPoll.pdf (accessed Dec. 1, 2007).

- Smith B: Test your stamina for workplace fatigue. *Nurs Manage* 35:38–40, Oct. 2004.

- Smith-Coggins R., et al.: Improving alertness and performance in emergency department physicians and nurses: The use of planned naps. *Ann Emerg Med* 48:596–604, Nov. 2006.

- Trinkoff A.M., et al.: Work schedule, needle use, and needlestick injuries among registered nurses. *Infect Control Hosp Epidemiol* 28:156–164, Feb. 2007.

Resources on Burnout

- Aiken L., et al.: Hospital nurse staffing and patient mortality, nurse burnout, and job satisfaction. *JAMA* 288:1987–1993, Oct. 2002.

- Cordes C., Dougherty T.: A review and an integration of research on job burnout. *Academy of Management Review* 18:621–656, Oct. 1993.

- Felton J.S.: Burnout as a clinical entity: Its importance in health care workers. *Occup Med (Lond)* 48:237–250, 1998.

- Maslach C.: Burned-out. *Human Behavior* 4:16–22, 1976.

- Maslach C., et al.: *Maslach Burnout Inventory,* 3rd ed. Palo Alto, CA: Consulting Psychologists Press, 1996.

- Medland J.: Fostering psychosocial wellness in oncology nurses: Addressing burnout and social support in the workplace. *Oncol Nurs Forum* 31:47–54, 2004.

- Penson R., et al.: Burnout: Caring for the caregivers. *Oncologist* 5:425–434, 2000.

Web Sites

Agency for Healthcare Research and Quality: http://www.ahrq.gov
American Academy of Sleep Medicine: http://www.aasmnet.org
American Council for Graduate Medical Education: http://www.acgme.org
American Society of Anesthesiologists: http://www.asahq.org
Centers for Disease Control and Prevention: http://www.cdc.gov
Helpguide (a project of the Center for Healthy Aging): http://www.helpguide.org
Institute for Healthcare Improvement: http://www.ihi.org
National Heart Lung and Blood Institute: http://www.nhlbi.nih.gov
National Institute for Occupational Safety and Health: http://www.cdc.gov/Niosh
National Sleep Foundation: http://www.sleepfoundation.org
VA National Center for Patient Safety: http://www.va.gov/NCPS

APPENDIX TWO

Effects of Health Care Provider Work Hours and Sleep Deprivation on Safety and Performance

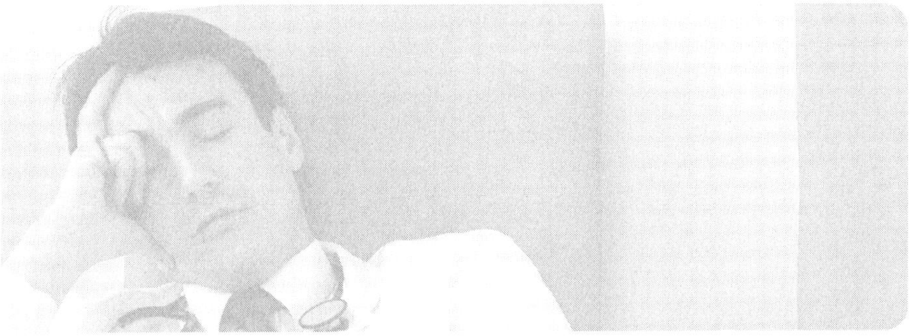

Steven W. Lockley, Ph.D.
Laura K. Barger, Ph.D.
Najib T. Ayas, M.D., M.P.H.
Jeffrey M. Rothschild, M.D., M.P.H.
Charles A. Czeisler, Ph.D., M.D.
Christopher P. Landrigan, M.D., M.P.H.
For the Harvard Work Hours, Health and Safety Group

During the past three years, a series of studies have demonstrated the risks to patients and providers of long work hours in health care. Compared with nurses working shorter hours, nurses working greater than 12.5–13 consecutive hours report (1): a 1.9- to 3.3-fold increased odds of making an error in patient care;[1,2] (2) a significantly increased risk of suffering a needlestick injury, exposing them to an increased risk of acquiring hepatitis, HIV, or other bloodborne illnesses;[3] and (3) significant decrease in vigilance on the job.[2]

Likewise, physicians-in-training working long hours have been found to be at greatly increased risk of injuring their patients or themselves. Recent research has demonstrated that physicians-in-training working traditional schedules with recurrent 24-hour shifts:

- Make 36% more serious medical errors than those whose scheduled work is limited to 16 consecutive hours[4]
- Make five times as many serious diagnostic errors[4]
- Have twice as many on-the-job attentional failures at night[5]
- Suffer 61% more needlestick and other sharp injuries after their 20th consecutive hour of work[6]

- Double their risk of a motor vehicle crash when driving home after 24 hours of work[7]
- Experience a 1.5 to 2 standard deviation (S.D.) deterioration in performance relative to baseline rested performance on both clinical and nonclinical tasks[8]
- Suffer decrements in performance commensurate with those induced by a blood alcohol level of 0.05 to 0.10%[9,10]
- Report making 300% more fatigue-related medical errors that lead to a patient's death[11]

In this article, we review these studies in detail and place these findings in the context of the biologic mechanisms known to underlie the development of fatigue. In the companion article by Landrigan et al.,[12] the manner in which these data have informed policy will be discussed, as will the need for evidence-based changes in current work- hour regulations.

Background: Sleep Deprivation and Circadian Misalignment

As the science of sleep and circadian medicine has advanced, the neurobiologic pathways that drive human performance and alertness have become better understood (Figure 1, page 115). We briefly discuss the state of the science regarding sleep and performance as it relates to health care workers and then discuss recent clinical studies that have directly assessed the effects of long work hours and sleep deprivation on physicians and nurses.

Circadian Rhythms

Health care providers regularly work during the biological night, when the endogenous drive for alertness is lowest. The endogenous circadian pacemaker, situated in the suprachiastmatic nuclei (SCN) of the hypothalamus, controls the intrinsic rhythms of sleep, alertness, and performance, among many other physiological and behavioral parameters, with the maximal drive for alertness emanating from the pacemaker during the biologic day, and maximal drive for sleepiness during the biologic night (Figure 1a).[13–15] Changes in work schedules from days to nights or from days off to nights are often too rapid to allow the circadian system to adapt to the scheduled wakefulness at night, placing many providers in a permanent state of "jet lag" as they attempt to remain awake and work, and subsequently sleep, at the incorrect internal circadian phase.[16,17] Such circadian misalignment is responsible for the higher rates of accidents by night-shift workers[18] and by drivers at night.[19]

Acute Sleep Deprivation

Nurses or physicians working nights after they have been awake during the day also

Figure 1.
Examples from Experimental Data Sets of the Four Major Physiologic Determinants of Fatigue

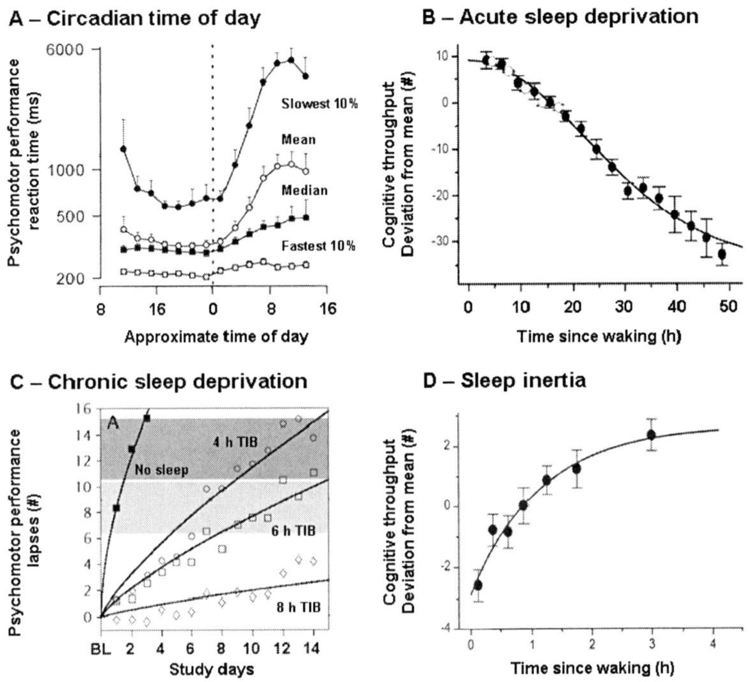

Figure 1a. *The figure shows examples from experimental data sets of the four major physiologic determinants of fatigue.*

Figure 1a illustrates the endogenous circadian rhythm in visual psychomotor performance (mean, median, 10% slowest, and 10% fastest responses) during a 32-hour vigil under constant conditions (n = 10). Performance is poorest towards the end of the biologic night but then improves again slightly, even in subjects remaining continually awake (although not equivalent to the same clock time 24 hours earlier because of the prolonged acute sleep deprivation) because of the drive for alertness emanating from the endogenous circadian pacemaker. Although average reaction times may slow to ~1 second, there is more than a 10-fold increase in the slowest 10% of responses, which average nearly 6 seconds at the circadian nadir before the subject reacts to a visual stimulus, which would represent a significant lapse of attention under real-world conditions. Reproduced with permission from Cajochen C., et al.: EEG and ocular correlates of circadian melatonin phase and human performance decrements during sleep loss. Am J Physiol Regul Integr Comp Physiol *277:R640–R649, Sep. 1999.*

(continued)

Figure 1. (continued)
Examples from Experimental Data Sets of the Four Major Physiologic Determinants of Fatigue

***Figure 1b** shows the effects of 48 hours of continual wakefulness on mean (± standard error of the mean[sem]) cognitive throughput, as measured by a simple 4-minute addition test in subjects measured under constant routine (●,* n = *147) or forced desynchrony (○,* n = *11) conditions. Cognition declines sigmoidally with increasing time awake. The line represents a model prediction of cognition under these conditions. Reproduced with permission from Jewett M.E., et al.: Sigmoidal decline of homeostatic component in subjective alertness and cognitive throughput.* Sleep *22(suppl.):S94–S95, Jun. 1999.*

***Figure 1c** shows how different amounts of chronic partial sleep deprivation affect psychomotor performance and compares the time course of average daily lapses in attention (based on 2-hourly tests from 7:30 A.M.–11:30 P.M.) during two weeks in subjects with an 8-hour (◇,* n = *9), 6-hour (□,* n = *13) and 4-hour (○,* n = *13) time-in-bed (TIB) sleep opportunity each day, and 88-hours of continuous sleep deprivation (■,* n *=13). Performance deteriorated in both the 6- and 4-hour sleep groups such that after 14 days, the 6-hour sleep group performed at an equivalent level to those kept awake for 24 hours continuously, and the 4-hour group was performing at the same level as someone kept awake for 3 whole days. Reproduced with permission from Dongen H.P., et al.: The cumulative cost of additional wakefulness: Dose-response effects on neurobehavioral functions and sleep physiology from chronic sleep restriction and total sleep deprivation.* Sleep *26:117–126, Mar. 2003. Erratum in:* Sleep *27:600, Jun. 15, 2004.*

***Figure 1d** shows the time course of sleep inertia in cognitive throughput during the first 4 hours of wakefulness after a normal 8-hour sleep for 3 days. Although there is an exponential improvement in performance over time, it takes at least 2 hours to reach maximal performance and there is a highest risk of a fatigue-related error in the first 30 minutes after waking. Reproduced with permission from Jewett M.E., et al.: Time course of sleep inertia dissipation in human performance and alertness.* J Sleep Res *8:1–8, Mar. 1999.*

Source: Joint Commission Resources, 2007.

suffer deterioration in performance because of long episodes of continuous wakefulness; residents working extended 24- to 30-hour on-duty shifts invariably experience these effects. Independent of the circadian system, acute continuous sleep deprivation has a profound impact on fatigue: After about 16–18 hours of wakefulness, alertness and performance decline rapidly (Figure 1b).[20,21] When prolonged wakefulness is coincident with being awake at an adverse circadian phase, for example, in the latter half of an extended-duration on-call shift, these two factors interact nonlinearly such that their combined effects exceed their individual decrements, making this a particularly critical and vulnerable time for the risk of a fatigue-related error or accident,[22,23] as we have demonstrated repeatedly in medical residents[4–7,11]

Chronic Partial Sleep Deprivation

Residents and nurses are also frequently exposed to chronic partial sleep deprivation, often for many months at a time, as they repeatedly fail to gain adequate sleep on a daily basis. Young adults would spontaneously sleep an average of approximately 8.5 hours per night if given sufficient opportunity, even following several nights of longer sleep.[24,25] Young adult residents working extended-duration shifts, however, sleep about 2 hours less than this amount on average per day,[5,26,27] guaranteeing a chronic buildup of sleep pressure. Nurses, particularly those who regularly work nights, also typically fail to achieve their average daily sleep requirements.[28] Repeated failure to gain sufficient sleep to fully recover from the previous wake episode has a cumulative detrimental effect on waking function that rapidly builds to significantly impair performance.[29,30] For example, after less than two weeks with only 6 hours time in bed per night, performance levels are equivalent to those observed after 24 hours of acute sleep deprivation, and after one week of only 4 hours in bed per night, performance is equivalent to that following 48 hours without sleep (Figure 1c).[30] Even more concerning for health care provider scheduling, however, is the disassociation between self-ratings of alertness and objective performance under such conditions.[30] Although performance continues to decline during several weeks of chronic partial sleep deprivation, subjective ratings level off, making self-assessment of fatigue and performance unreliable, much in the same way that occurs following alcohol consumption. Institution-level protections to ensure adequate alertness on duty are required, therefore, rather than relying on individual self-policing of fatigue.

Sleep Inertia

A fourth factor that can affect performance is the phenomenon of sleep inertia, the impairment present immediately on awakening from sleep. Naps during residents' on-duty shifts have been tested as a countermeasure to chronic and acute sleep deprivation.[31,32] Although these may be beneficial in ameliorating performance decrements following a period of recovery, such naps, which are often taken under very high levels of sleep pressure, can induce postnap impairment. Alertness and performance are not maximal immediately on waking, and it takes several hours to realize a fully alert state (Figure 1d).[33] Sleep inertia dissipates exponentially, but the first 15–30 minutes after waking are a particularly vulnerable period. Performance decrements at this time can exceed those experiences after 24 hours of continuous wakefulness (Figure 2, on page 118).[34] Requiring residents and nurses to make vital decisions shortly after being woken on duty therefore presents a very high risk of fatigue-related error.

Figure 2.
Examples from Experimental Data Sets of the Four Major Physiologic Determinants of Fatigue

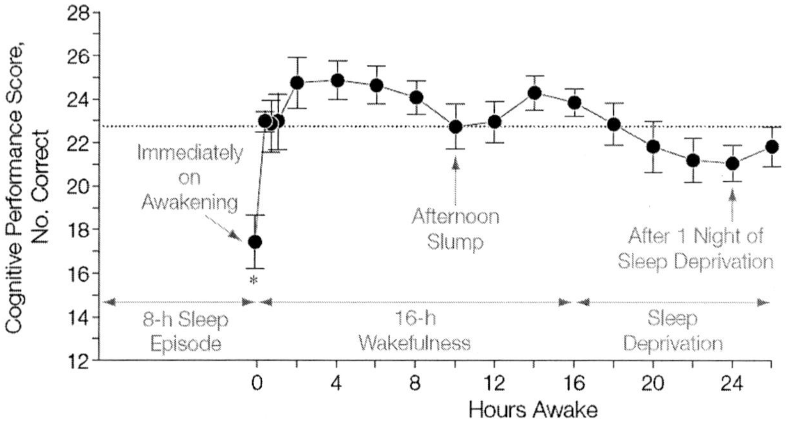

*The figure shows the relative impact of sleep inertia and acute sleep deprivation on cognitive performance (*n = *9: 8 men, 1 woman, 20–41 years of age). After 6 days with an 8-hour sleep opportunity at the same time each night, subjects remained awake for 26 hours under constant conditions and completed a simple addition task at ~1, 21, 41, and 61 minutes after awakening, and then every 2 hours. Cognitive performance was worst immediately after waking and more impaired than following 24 hours of continuous wakefulness. These data highlight the particular risk of residents committing a fatigue-related error when woken from sleep on duty by a page. Reproduced with permission from Wertz A.T., et al.: Effects of sleep inertia on cognition.* JAMA *295:163–164, Jan. 11, 2006. Copyright ©2006 American Medical Association.*

Source: Joint Commission Resources, 2007.

Sleep Deprivation and Learning

In addition to the immediate effects on clinicians' alertness and performance (discussed in the section, "Recent Clinical Studies"), long-term adverse effects of sleep deprivation are increasingly being recognized. Particularly relevant both to medical trainees and junior nurses is the impact of sleep and sleep deprivation on learning and memory.[35–37] Many tasks, including visual discrimination, motor learning, and insight are dependent on adequate sleep following the initial learning opportunity,[37–40] and failure to sleep the night after learning a task may impair providers' ability to consolidate this learning.[40,41]

Sleep Deprivation and Health

There are also longer-term health detriments due to shift work and chronic sleep deprivation. Sleep deprivation and the circadian system affect metabolic processes,[42–44] which may result in increased risk of cardiovascular disease, insulin resistance, and diabetes.[45] Regular night-shift workers also have a increased risk of certain cancers, particularly breast cancer, as compared with non-shift workers.[46,47] Resident schedules are among the most extreme of any profession and may present even greater risks than standard night-shift work.

Recent Clinical Studies: Health Care Provider Sleep Deprivation, Performance, and Safety

Although an extensive literature on sleep deprivation, circadian misalignment, and human performance has accrued during the past three decades, debate on the effects of these factors on physicians and nurses has persisted. The notion that providers' long work hours might have an adverse effect on their performance and safety is not new. More than 35 years ago, it was recognized that extended work hours adversely affect medical[48,49] and surgical[50] performance. Subsequent studies have also documented additional adverse effects on provider health and well- being.[51–54] The importance of these effects in clinical (as opposed to simulated or laboratory) settings, however, was previously somewhat unclear. Consequently, we and others initiated a series of studies during the past several years on the effects of sleep deprivation on provider performance and patient and provider safety.

Effect of the Extended Work Hours of Physicians-in-Training on Physician-in-Training Safety: The HWHHS National Cohort Study

In 2001, concerned with the potential risks of residents' extended duty hours on the safety of patients and providers, we formed the Harvard Work Hours, Health, and Safety (HWHHS) Group, an interdisciplinary collaboration between investigators interested in rigorously evaluating the effects of provider sleep deprivation on safety. With the support of the Agency for Healthcare Research and Quality (AHRQ) and the National Institute of Occupational Safety and Health (NIOSH), we began a prospective nationwide Web-based survey of 2,737 postgraduate year (PGY)-1 residents (53% female, mean age ± S.D. = 28.0 ± 3.9 yrs) in 2002 (a year before publication of the Accreditation Council for Graduate Medical Education (ACGME) guidelines on duty hours) to examine the impact of extended-duration work hours on resident health and patient safety.

Methods. Most participants were medical residents (79%), with 11% from surgical programs and 10% in other or nonspecified specialties; 85% were graduates of medical schools in the United States. Volunteers completed a total of 17,003 monthly reports between June 2002 and May 2003 that included questions about their work hours, sleep, motor vehicle crashes, occupational injuries and self-reported medical errors among approximately 60 questions.[6,7,11] Monthly sleep and work hour reports were validated by daily diaries for three to four weeks in 7% of the cohort using the same methods that we have shown to be highly correlated ($r \geq 0.98$) with continuous observation and polysomnographically determined sleep, respectively.[5] The number of work hours reported on the survey per month (mean ± S.D. = 249.8 ± 75.3 h) correlated with the daily work hour diaries (244.0 ± 69.3 h; $r = 0.76$, $p < .001$, $n = 192$), and the number of extended shifts reported by the two methods (3.6 ± 3.3 and 3.5 ± 2.8, respectively; $r = 0.94$, $p < .001$, $n = 40$).[7]

Additional information was requested in support of the reported motor vehicle accidents and percutaneous injuries. A police report, insurance claim, repair record or photograph of the damaged vehicle, medical record, or written description of the crash was obtained for 82% of all reported motor vehicle crashes. Respondents reporting occupational exposure to body fluids were asked about the type of exposure, the location and time of exposure, whether it was formally reported, the number of hours worked prior to the exposure, and the cause(s) of the exposure. Only percutaneous injuries due to a needlestick or cut with another sharp instrument for which the location and time of the incident were provided were included in analysis. Similar follow-up details were requested for self-reported medical errors.

PGY-1 residents reported completing extended-duration work shifts (> 24 h) an average (± S.D.) of 3.9 ± 3.4 times per month, with a mean duration of each extended-duration work shift of 32.0 ± 0.7 hours. Sleep was minimal on these shifts, averaging 3.2 (± 1.6) and 2.6 (± 1.7) hours for those with and without night-float coverage, respectively. The mean maximal hours of continuous wakefulness reported on these shifts was 25.3 ± 8.3 hours.[7]

Using a within-person case-crossover design, we assessed the number and proportion of motor vehicle crashes and near-miss incidents that occurred following an extended-duration work shift, compared with those following a nonextended shift for each subject.[7] We also calculated the rate of percutaneous injuries that occurred during the day following an on-call overnight extended shift with the same clock time (6:30 A.M.–5:30 A.M.) the day before for each subject, and separately compared daytime (7:30 A.M.–3:30 P.M.) and night-time (11:30 P.M.–7:30 A.M.) injury rates.[6] Finally, the rate of self-reported medical errors and attentional failures was similarly calculated for months with one to four or five or more extended-duration work shifts and compared within-subjects to months without such shifts.[11]

Results. Figure 3 on page 121 shows the rate of motor vehicle crashes, near-misses accidents, and percutanous injuries in relation to extended-duration work shifts.

Figure 3.
Residents' Motor Vehicle Crashes, Near-Miss Motor Vehicle Accidents, and Percutaneous Injuries Reported Relative to the Duration of Work Shifts

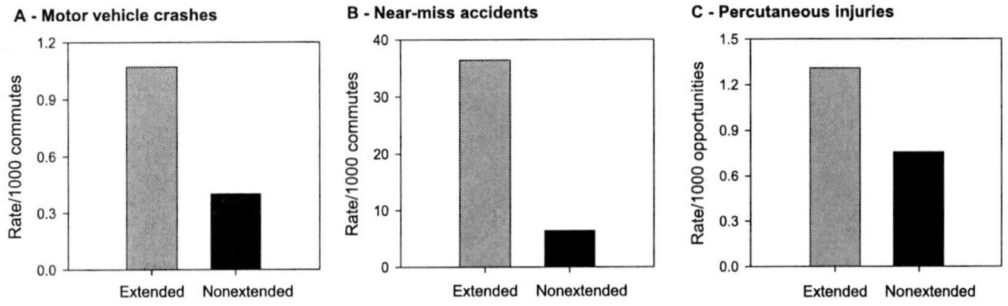

This figure shows the rate of (A) motor vehicle crashes, (B) near-miss motor vehicle accidents and (C) percutaneous injuries reported by postgraduate year (PGY)-1 residents nationwide (n = 2,737) in 17,007 monthly reports between June 2002 and May 2003 relative to the duration of work shifts. Residents reported a significantly higher rate of motor vehicle crashes and near misses on the commute following an extended-duration work shift (> 24 hours; Figures A and B, ■) as compared with the same residents' commute following a nonextended shift (< 24 hours, ■). The Mantel–Haenszel odds ratios (OR ± 95% confidence interval) for having an accident or near miss on the commute home were 2.3 (1.6–3.3) and 5.9 (5.4–6.3), respectively (see text). Residents also reported a significantly higher rate of percutaneous injuries when on duty during the day after being on-call overnight (6:30-17:30; Figure C, ■) as compared with the day before on-call (■; OR 1.61, 1.46–1.78).

Figures A and B: Data replotted from Barger L.K., et al.: Extended work shifts and the risk of motor vehicle crashes among interns. N Engl J Med *352:125–134, Jan. 13, 2005.*

Figure C: Data replotted with permission from Ayas N.T., et al.: Extended work duration and the risk of self-reported percutaneous injuries in interns. JAMA *296:1055–1062, Sep. 6, 2006. Copyright ©2006 American Medical Association.*

Source: Joint Commission Resources, 2007.

The associated Mantel-Haenszel odds ratios (odds ratio [OR] ± 95% confidence limit) for a crash on the commute after an extended shift was 2.3 (1.6–3.3; $p < .001$) and 5.9 (5.4–6.3) for a near miss ($p < .001$), as compared with the commute after a nonextended shift (OR = 1.0). There was a linear relationship between the number of extended shifts per month and the subsequent occurrence of crashes such that each extended-duration work shift increased (1) the rate of any crash by an additional 9.1% (3.4%–14.7%) over baseline and (2) the risk of a crash on the commute from work by 16.2% (7.8%–24.7%).[7]

The odds of suffering a percutaneous injury between 6:30–17:30 after working overnight was 1.61 (1.46–1.78), as compared with the same times on the previous day.[6] The primary reasons attributed to the injury by the residents were a lapse in concentration (64%), fatigue (31%), leaving a sharp exposed (18%), patient movement (17%), and inadequate lighting (7%). Of note, only 58% of the injuries were reported to the residents' occupational health services. There was also a significant difference between injury rates by time of day; the odds of suffering a percutaneous injury at night were twice that during the day (OR 2.04, 1.98–2.11).

Effect of Nurses' Extended Work Hours on Nurses' Safety

In a similar evaluation of the association between nurses' working conditions and needlestick injuries, Trinkoff and colleagues conducted a longitudinal survey of 2,273 nurses between November 2002 and April 2004.[3] Overall, 16.3% of respondents reported having suffered a needlestick injury. The number of needles nurses estimated using each day was significantly associated with the odds of injury. In addition, hours worked per day, weekends worked per month, working evening and night shifts, and working 13 or more hours per day at least once per week were each significantly associated with needlestick injuries. The authors concluded that nurses' extended work schedules increased the incidence of needlestick injuries and that work hour reductions could reduce needlestick injuries.

Effect of Resident-Physicians' Extended Work Hours on Patient Safety: The HWHHS National Cohort Study

In the HWHHS study, the rate of self-reported fatigue-related medical errors, including those that resulted in a preventable adverse patient outcome or patient fatality, also increased with the increasing number of extended-duration work shifts per month (Figure 4, page 123). Conversely, medical errors reported not to be fatigue related were not dependent on the number of extended-duration shifts. The odd ratios of reporting a medical error were 3.5 (3.3–3.7) and 7.5 (7.2–7.8) when working one to four or more than five extended-duration shifts per month, respectively, as compared with those months without extended work shifts. For adverse events, the odds were 8.7 (3.4–22) and 7.0 (4.3–11), respectively. The odds ratio of reporting a fatigue-related fatality was only significantly higher when working five or more extended shifts per month (4.1, 1.4–12). These rates were not affected by age or gender. Similar relationships between errors and the number of extended

Figure 4.
Medical Errors Reported by Residents Relative to the Number of Extended-Duration Work Shifts (> 24 hours) per Month

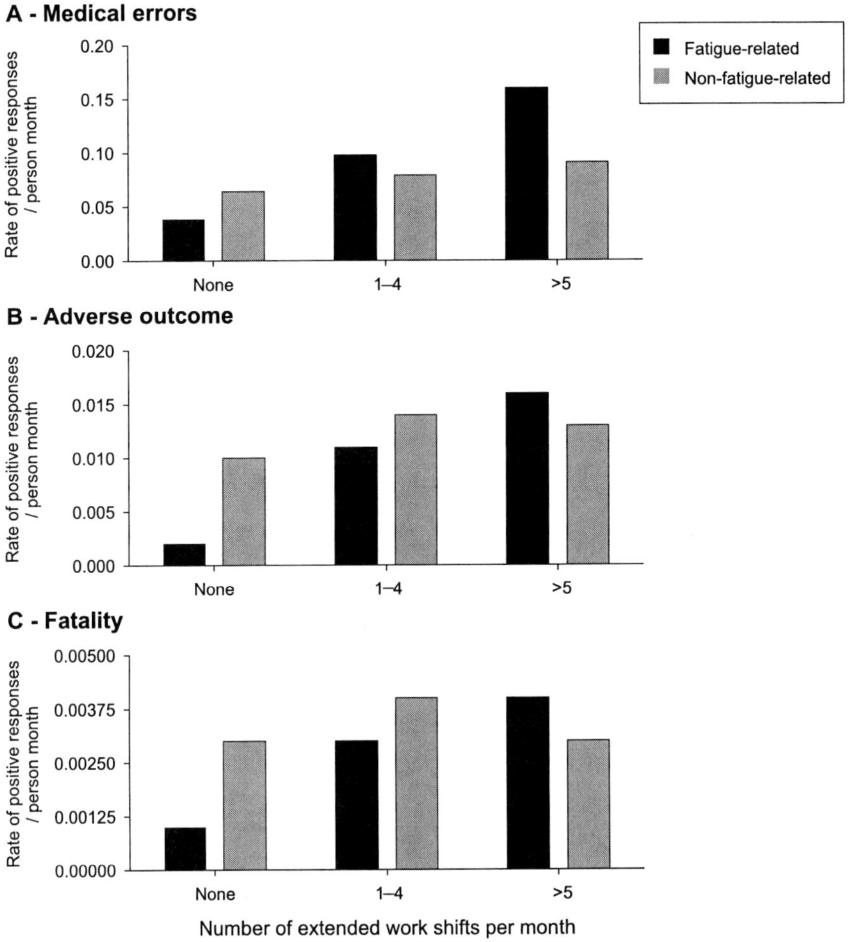

This figure shows the rate of (A) medical errors, (B) medical errors resulting in an adverse patient outcome and (C) medical errors resulting in a patient fatality reported by post-graduate year (PGY)-1 residents relative to the number of extended-duration work shifts (> 24 hours) worked per month and whether the resident ascribed the error as fatigue-

(continued)

Figure 4. (continued)
Medical Errors Reported by Residents Relative to the Number of Extended-Duration Work Shifts (> 24 hours) per Month

related (■) or non-fatigue-related (■). The rate of self-reported fatigue-related errors increased with increasing number of extended-duration shifts. The odds ratios (OR ± 95% confidence interval) for medical errors, adverse outcomes, and fatalities in months when residents worked five or more extended-duration shifts were 7.5 (7.2–7.8), 7.0 (4.3–11), and 4.1 (1.4–12), respectively, as compared with months in which no extended-duration shifts were reported (see text). The rate of self-reported errors not categorized as due to fatigue did not increase significantly with the number of extended-duration shifts. Data replotted from Barger L.K., et al.: Impact of extended-duration shifts on medical errors, adverse events, and attentional failures. PLoS Med *3:e487, Dec. 2006.*

Source: Joint Commission Resources, 2007.

shifts were observed in residents who completed all monthly surveys and when analyses were limited to hospital wards only, suggesting no major effects of reporting bias or patient acuity.[11]

The probability of reporting an attentional failure while on duty or during educational activities was also related to the number of extended shifts worked. The odds of reporting falling asleep during surgery were 2.1 (1.7–2.7) and 1.4 (1.3–1.6) for one to four or five or more extended shifts, respectively, and 1.5 (1.3–1.7) and 2.1 (2.0–2.2) for falling asleep during a patient examination. Higher rates of falling asleep during attending rounds and during lectures were also reported, with ORs of 5.5 (5.4–5.7) and 4.3 (4.3–4.4), respectively, when working five or more extended shifts per month. Consistent with these results, the reported sleep duration decreased with increasing numbers of extended shifts worked per month. Residents reported sleeping on average (± S.D.) 179.3 (± 54.3) hours per month when not working extended shifts, 176.6 (± 45.1) hours when working one to four extended shifts per month, and 165.3 (± 39.2) when working five or more per month.[11]

Effect of Nurses' Extended Work Hours on Patient Safety

In two separate studies, Rogers, Scott, and colleagues have demonstrated that nurses working greater than 12.5 consecutive hours are at significantly increased risk of making a medical error. In the first study, 393 randomly selected members of the American Nurses Association logged their work hours daily and reported all medical errors in which they were involved; data were collected on a total of 5,317 work shifts.[1] Thirty-nine percent of all shifts exceeded 12.5 hours, and working ≥ 12.5 hours was associated with a threefold increased risk (OR = 3.29, $p = .001$) of making an error.

In the second study, Scott et al. conducted a similar evaluation of a random sample of nurses drawn from the membership of the American Association of Critical-Care Nurses.[2] In this study of 502 nurses and 6,017 work shifts, it was found that 67% of critical care nurses' work shifts exceeded 12 hours and that working 16-hour shifts was common. Nurses working more than 12.5 hours had twice the risk of making a medical error (OR = 1.94, $p = .03$).

Effect of Resident-Physicians' Extended Work Hours on Resident Alertness and Patient Safety: The Intern Sleep and Patient Safety Study

At the same time that the HWHHS National Cohort Study was launched, we initiated a prospective, randomized trial to test the effect of eliminating extended-duration work shifts in two critical care units on resident sleep and fatigue and the rate of serious medical errors. Because this was designed principally as a randomized intervention trial, it is discussed in detail in the companion article by Landrigan et al.[12] regarding implementation of work-hour limits. With respect to the current review of the effects of long work hours on safety, however, it is relevant to mention here that in addition to demonstrating the effectiveness of reducing interns' work hours as a means of improving patient safety, this study demonstrated in a clinical setting that provider sleep deprivation leads to significantly impaired alertness and increased rates of medical errors. Interns working a traditional schedule with frequent 24–30 hour shifts had twice the rate of electrooculogram-derived attentional failures[5] (traditional: 0.69 ± 0.13/hour; intervention: 0.33 ± 0.09/hour; $p < .02$) than they had when working an intervention schedule that limited their scheduled work to 16 consecutive hours. In addition, they made 35.9% more serious medical errors than when the same residents worked the intervention schedule (traditional: 136.0/1000 patient days; intervention: 100.1/1000 patient days; $p < 0.001$), including more than five times more serious diagnostic errors during the traditional as compared with the intervention schedule.[4]

Physician Sleep Deprivation and Impairment: Comparison of the Effects of a Traditional On-Call Schedule and Alcohol

During the past decade, several studies have compared the level of cognitive impairment due to sleep deprivation with that caused by alcohol and have shown that performance after being awake for 24 hours or more is equivalent to that of someone who is legally drunk.[9] In a recent study that specifically tested 34 PGY1–PGY3 residents, psychomotor performance reaction, commission errors, and lane and speed variability on a driving simulator and subjective alertness were as impaired following four weeks of "heavy" call rotation (~90 hours per week, including 34–36 hours continuous duty every fourth or fifth night, during which residents obtained an average of 3 hours of sleep per night when on duty) as following a month of "light" call (~44 hours/week and night-call only under emergency circumstances) plus moderate alcohol intake 20 minutes before the testing sessions (~0.05 g% blood alcohol concentration).[10]

Physician Impairment and Clinical Tasks: A Meta-Analysis

In an effort to pull together all the studies conducted during the past three decades on physician and nonphysician performance and sleep deprivation, Philibert conducted a recent meta-review on behalf of ACGME.[8] In this analysis, 60 studies of the effects of sleep deprivation and fatigue on both physicians and nonphysicians were reviewed. On meta-analysis, it was found that continuous duty of 24–30 hours reduced overall performance by nearly one S.D. and reduced physicians' clinical performance by more than 1.5 S.D. (Figure 5, page 127).

Conclusion

Collectively, the weight of current evidence strongly suggests that extended-duration work shifts significantly increase fatigue and impair performance. Residents' traditional work shifts of 24–30 consecutive hours unquestionably increase the risk of serious medical errors and diagnostic mistakes and have been shown in a national cohort study to increase the risk of harmful and fatal medical errors. Nursing shifts of more than 12.5 hours are common and similarly appear to greatly increase the risk of medical error. Likewise, long work hours increase the risk that nurses and doctors will suffer an occupational injury with potentially devastating long-term consequences and increase the risk of motor vehicle crashes, a leading cause of mortality among young adults. Thus, both from the standpoint of providers and patients, the hours routinely worked by health care providers in the United States are unsafe.

As Landrigan et al.[12] discuss, governments abroad have taken an active stance to address this problem. To reduce the unacceptably high rate of preventable fatigue-related medical error and injury among health care workers, the United States must establish and enforce safe work-hour limits for health care providers.

Figure 5.
Effect of 24–30 Hours of Acute Sleep Loss on Various Types of Performance Based on a Meta-Analysis of 60 Sleep-Deprivation Studies of Physicians and Nonphysicians

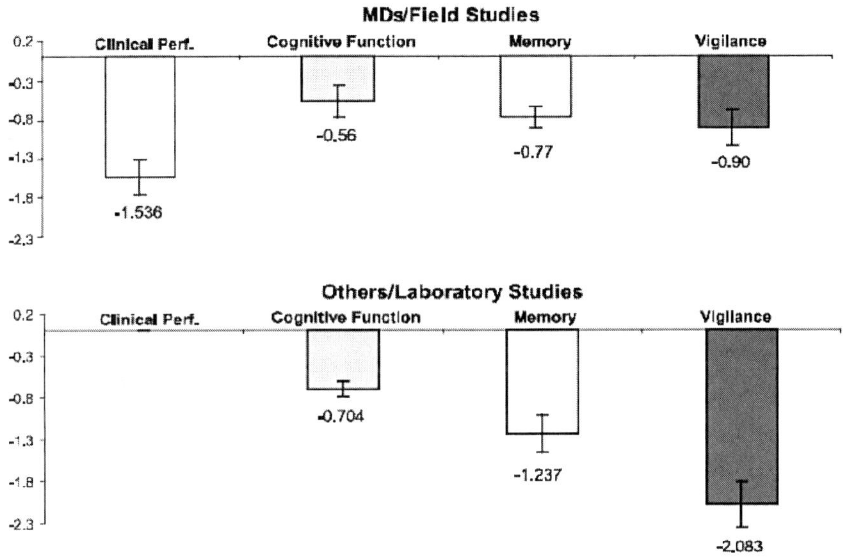

The figure shows the effect of 24–30 hours of acute sleep loss on various types of performance based on a meta-analysis of 60 sleep-deprivation studies of physicians (top panel) and nonphysicians (bottom panel). The average effect sizes are shown for each performance type and are corrected for measurement error and standard error of the corrected effect sizes. Following 24–30 hours on duty, physicians' clinical performance deteriorated by ~ 1.5 standard deviations as compared to when 'rested' (top panel). As most of these data were collected under 'field' conditions, however, physicians in the 'rested' condition were unlikely to be non-fatigued, which may explain the greater effect of sleep deprivation observed under more highly controlled laboratory conditions (bottom panel). Reproduced with permission from Philibert I.: Sleep loss and performance in residents and nonphysicians: A meta-analytic examination. Sleep *28(11):1392–1402, Nov. 1, 2005.*

Source: Joint Commission Resources, 2007.

The authors thank the members of the Harvard Work Hours, Health and Safety Group: Daniel Aeschbach, Ph.D.; David E. Bates, M.D.; Elizabeth Burdick, M.S.; Brian E. Cade, M.S.; John W. Cronin, M.D.; Erin E. Evans, R.P.S.G.T.; Joel T. Katz, M.D.; Rainu Kaushal, M.D., M.P.H.; Clark J. Lee, J.D.; Craig M. Lilly, M.D.; Bernard Rosner, Ph.D.; Jeffrey M. Rothschild, M.D., M.P.H.; Frank E. Speizer, M.D.; and Peter H. Stone, M.D.

The work of the Harvard Work Hours, Health, and Safety Group discussed in this manuscript has been supported by grants from the Agency for Healthcare Research and Quality (U18 HS015906 and RO1 HS12032), affording data confidentiality protection by federal statute (Public Health Service Act; 42 U.S.C.), the National Institute for Occupational Safety and Health within the U.S. Centers for Disease Control (R01 OH07567), which provided a Certificate of Confidentiality for data protection; and Brigham and Women's Hospital. Dr. Landrigan is the recipient of an AHRQ career development award (K08 HS13333), and Dr. Barger was the recipient of a National Heart, Lung, and Blood Institute fellowship in the program of training in Sleep, Circadian, and Respiratory Neurobiology at Brigham and Women's Hospital (NHLBI; T32 HL079010). Dr. Czeisler is supported in part by the Air Force Office of Scientific Research and by the National Space Biomedical Research Institute through the National Aeronautics and Space Administration (NCC9-58).

This article originally appeared in The Joint Commission Journal on Quality and Patient Safety, November 2007, vol. 33, No. 11 Supplement.

References

1. Rogers A.E., et al.: The working hours of hospital staff nurses and patient safety. *Health Aff (Millwood)* 23:202–212, Jul.–Aug. 2004.

2. Scott L.D., et al.: Effects of critical care nurses' work hours on vigilance and patients' safety. *Am J Crit Care* 15:30–37, Jan. 2006.

3. Trinkoff A.M., et al.: Work schedule, needle use, and needlestick injuries among registered nurses. *Infect Control Hosp Epidemiol* 28:156–164, Feb. 2007.

4. Landrigan C.P., et al.: Effect of reducing interns' work hours on serious medical errors in intensive care units. *N Engl J Med* 351:1838–1848, Oct. 28, 2004.

5. Lockley S.W., et al.: Effect of reducing interns' weekly work hours on sleep and attentional failures. *N Engl J Med* 351:1829–1837, Oct. 28, 2004.

6. Ayas N.T., et al.: Extended work duration and the risk of self-reported percutaneous injuries in interns. *JAMA* 296:1055–1062, Sep. 6, 2006.

7. Barger L.K., et al.: Extended work shifts and the risk of motor vehicle crashes among interns. *N Engl J Med* 352:125–134, Jan. 13, 2005.

8. Philibert I.: Sleep loss and performance in residents and nonphysicians: A meta-analytic examination. *Sleep* 28:1392–1402, Nov. 2005.

9. Dawson D., Reid K.: Fatigue, alcohol and performance impairment. *Nature* 388:235, Jul. 17, 1997.

10. Arnedt J.T., et al.: Neurobehavioral performance of residents after heavy night call vs. after alcohol ingestion. *JAMA* 294:1025–1033, Sep. 7, 2005.

11. Barger L.K., et al.: Impact of extended-duration shifts on medical errors, adverse events, and attentional failures. *PLoS Med* 3:e487, Dec. 2006.

12. Landrigan C.P., et al.: Effective implementation of work hour limits and systemic improvements. *Jt Comm J Qual Patient Saf* 33(suppl.):19–29, Nov. 2007.

13. Johnson M.P., et al.: Short-term memory, alertness and performance: A reappraisal of their relationship to body temperature. *J Sleep Res* 1:24–29, Mar. 1992.

14. Cajochen C., et al.: EEG and ocular correlates of circadian melatonin phase and human performance decrements during sleep loss. *Am J Physiol Regul Integr Comp Physiol* 277:R640–R649, Sep. 1999.

15. Monk T.H., et al.: Circadian determinants of subjective alertness. *J Biol Rhythms* 4:393-404, Winter 1989.

16. Czeisler C.A., et al.: Human sleep: Its duration and organization depend on its circadian phase. *Science* 210:1264–1267, Dec. 12, 1980.

17. Dijk D.J., Czeisler C.A.: Contribution of the circadian pacemaker and the sleep homeostat to sleep propensity, sleep structure, electroencephalographic slow waves, and sleep spindle activity in humans. *J Neurosci* 15:3526–3538, May 1995.

18. Folkard S., Tucker P.: Shift work, safety and productivity. *Occup Med (Lond)* 53:95–101, Mar. 2003.

19. National Highway Traffic Safety Administration: *Traffic Safety Facts 1999: A Compilation of Motor Vehicle Crash Data from the Fatality Analysis Reporting System and the General Estimates System.* Washington, DC: U.S. Department of Transportation, 2000.

20. Jewett M.E.: Models of Circadian and Homeostatic Regulation of Human Performance and Alertness (Ph.D. diss.). Harvard University, 1997.

21. Jewett M.E., Kronauer R.E.: Interactive mathematical models of subjective alertness and cognitive throughput in

humans. *J Biol Rhythms* 14:588–597, Dec. 1999.

22. Cajochen C., et al.: Non-linear interaction between the circadian and homeostatic modulation of slow eye movements during wakefulness in humans. *J Sleep Res* 9:58, 2000 [abstract].

23. Dijk D.J., Lockley S.W.: Integration of human sleep-wake regulation and circadian rhythmicity. *J Appl Physiol* 92:852–862, Feb. 2002.

24. Wehr T.A., et al.: Conservation of photoperiod-responsive mechanisms in humans. *Am J Physiol* 265:R846–R857, Oct. 1993.

25. Rajaratnam S.M., et al.: Melatonin advances the circadian timing of EEG sleep and directly facilitates sleep without altering its duration in extended sleep opportunities in humans. *J Physiol Regul Integr Comp Physiol* 561(pt. 1):339–351, Nov. 15, 2004.

26. Baldwin D.C. Jr., Daugherty S.R.: Sleep deprivation and fatigue in residency training: Results of a national survey of first-and second-year residents. *Sleep* 27:217–223, Mar. 2004.

27. Rosen I.M., et al.: Evolution of sleep quantity, sleep deprivation, mood disturbances, empathy, and burnout among interns. *Acad Med* 81:82–85, Jan. 2006.

28. Gold D.R., et al.: Rotating shift work, sleep, and accidents related to sleepiness in hospital nurses. *Am J Public Health* 82:1011–1014, Jul. 1992.

29. Belenky G., et al.: Patterns of performance degradation and restoration during sleep restriction and subsequent recovery: A sleep dose-response study. *J Sleep Res* 12:1–12, Mar. 2003.

30. Van Dongen H.P.A., et al.: The cumulative cost of additional wakefulness: Dose-response effects on neurobehavioral functions and sleep physiology from chronic sleep restriction and total sleep deprivation. *Sleep* 26:117–126, Mar. 15, 2003. Erratum in *Sleep* 27:600, Jun. 15, 2004.

31. Smith-Coggins R., et al.: Improving alertness and performance in emergency department physicians and nurses: The use of planned naps. *Ann Emerg Med* 48:596–604, Nov., 2006.

32. Arora V., et al.: The effects of on-duty napping on intern sleep time and fatigue. *Ann Intern Med* 144:792–798, Jun. 6, 2006.

33. Jewett M.E., et al.: Time course of sleep inertia dissipation in human performance and alertness. *J Sleep Res* 8:1–8, Mar. 1999.

34. Wertz A.T., et al.: Effects of sleep inertia on cognition. *JAMA* 295:163–164, Jan. 11, 2006.

35. Durmer J.S., Dinges D.F.: Neurocognitive consequences of sleep deprivation. *Semin Neurol* 25:117–129, Mar. 2005.

36. Ellenbogen J.M.: Cognitive benefits of sleep and their loss due to sleep deprivation. *Neurology* 64:E25–E27, Apr. 12, 2005.

37. Stickgold R.: Sleep-dependent memory consolidation. *Nature* 437:1272–1278, Oct. 27, 2005.

38. Wagner U., et al.: Sleep inspires insight. *Nature* 427:352–355, Jan. 22, 2004.

39. Walker M.P., et al.: Practice with sleep makes perfect: sleep-dependent motor skill learning. *Neuron* 35:205–211, Jul. 3, 2002.

40. Walker M.P., Stickgold R.: Sleep-dependent learning and memory consolidation. *Neuron* 44:121–133, Sep. 30, 2004.

41. Huber R., et al.: Local sleep and learning. *Nature* 430:78–81, Jul. 1, 2004.

42. Spiegel K., et al.: Sleep loss: A novel risk factor for insulin resistance and Type 2 diabetes. *J Appl Physiol* 99:2008–2019, Nov. 2005.

43. Hampton S.M., et al.: Postprandial hormone and metabolic responses in simulated shift work. *J Endocrinol* 151:259–267, Nov. 1996.

44. Ribeiro D., et al.: Altered postprandial hormone and metabolic responses in a simulated shift work environment. *J Endocrinol* 158:305–310, Sep. 1998.

45. Knutsson A.: Health disorders of shift workers. *Occup Med (Lond)* 53:103–108, Mar. 2003.

46. Davis S., Mirick D.K., Stevens R.G.: Night shift work, light at night, and risk of breast cancer. *J Natl Cancer Inst* 93:1557–1562, Oct. 17, 2001.

47. Schernhammer E.S., et al.: Rotating night shifts and risk of breast cancer in women participating in the nurses' health study. *J Natl Cancer Inst* 93:1563–1568, Oct. 17, 2001.

48. Friedman R.C., Bigger J.T., Kornfield D.S.: The intern and sleep loss. *N Engl J Med* 285:201–203, Jul. 22, 1971.

49. Friedman R.C., Kornfeld D.S., Bigger T.J.: Psychological problems associated with sleep deprivation in interns. *Journal of Medical Education* 48:436–441, May 1973.

50. Goldman L.I., McDonough M.T., Rosemond G.P.: Stresses affecting surgical performance and learning: I. Correlation of heart rate, electrocardiogram, and operation simultaneously recorded on videotapes. *J Surg Res* 12:83–86, Feb. 1972.

51. Ford C.V., Wentz D.K.: The internship year: A study of sleep, mood states, and psychophysiologic parameters. *South Med J* 77:1435–1442, Nov. 1984.

52. Reuben D.B.: Depressive symptoms in medical house officers. *Arch Intern Med* 145:286–288, Feb. 1985.

53. Steele M.T., et al.: The occupational risk of motor vehicle collisions for emergency medicine residents. *Acad Emerg Med* 6:1050–1053, Oct. 1999.

54. Parks D.K., et al.: Day-night pattern in accidental exposures to blood-borne pathogens among medical students and residents. *Chronobiol Int* 17:61–70, Jan. 2000.

APPENDIX THREE

The Change Calendar: A Tool to Prevent Change Fatigue

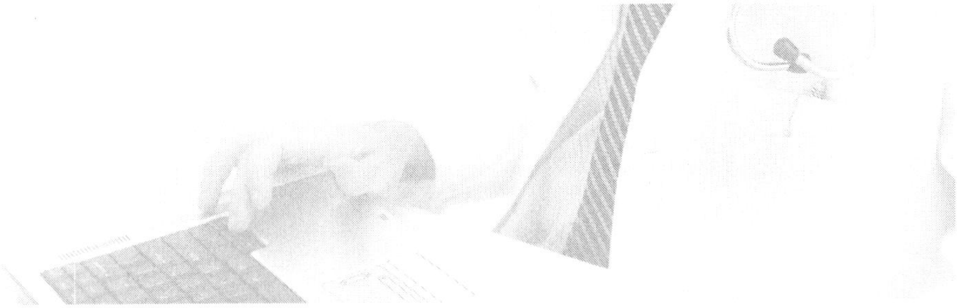

Direct and indirect care providers in complex health care settings are consistently challenged by environmental, human, and cognitive factors that inherently bring risk for error. When coupled with the avalanche of changes in process, equipment, and systems that care providers regularly experience, these factors take on even greater magnitude and set the stage for an even greater risk of error. Change management can be used to reduce that risk and create stability at the point of care delivery.

This article is not about leadership or cultural aspects of change management,[1] nor does it provide a review of change literature related to patient safety. It does provide a tool to help manage change at the operational level.

Change fatigue refers to impairments in an individual's and organization's abilities to cope with the ever-increasing scope and pace of change.[2] This article addresses the cumulative effect of multiple simultaneous changes and a strategy—use of the change calendar—to mitigate that effect. As Scott-Morgan et al. have stated: "Each oscillation in and out of stability disrupts the organization, leading to cumulative change fatigue...Companies should not fixate on change; they should concentrate on maximizing stability."[3 (p. xii)]

To address change in the context of change fatigue as a root cause of patient safety issues, management strategy and tactics must result in a process that "smooths" change by doing the following:

- Accurately forecast changes that affect caregivers
- Accurately assess the degree of impact of each change
- Proactively schedule changes on any given unit on any given week

Although the concept and objectives of "smoothing" change are simple, accomplishing those objectives can be difficult if the organization allows them to be.

Tool Description

The Change Calendar is a simple approach to manage the timing of any change that affects direct and indirect caregivers. It uses a weekly time line to inventory, evaluate, and coordinate a variety of changes occurring within units and across the organization. The Change Calendar is intended to proactively assess and schedule changes across the organization and to subsequently reduce the amount of distraction and change fatigue.

Tool Application to Safety

Health care is a decision-intensive industry, with frontline employees empowered to make high-risk decisions throughout an entire shift of duty. In such decision-intense environments, cognitive factors such as the following are often identified as contributing to error:

- Stress and fatigue
- Lack of familiarity with the task
- Trying something new under pressure
- Information overload
- Work load and multitasking
- Doing more with less resources
- Favoring production over safety
- Task saturation
- Task prioritization[4]

When these factors are combined with the volume and intensity of changes faced by the caregivers in health care organizations, the cumulative effect signals an increased potential for error.

Caregivers at the "sharp end" frequently express concern about the simultaneous implementation of uncoordinated changes.[5]

Reducing change fatigue should have a positive effect on the cognitive factors listed above. The Change Calendar can be used to help an organization make the transition from the current periodic "avalanche" to the future "snowfall" (Figure 1, on page 135). The drivers that accumulate to create the amount of change in an organization include not only strategic and tactical organizational changes (for example, implementation of an electronic medical record, new patient flow tracking and measurement) but also unit-specific changes (for example, core competency training, new nurse preceptoring).

Tool Application Setting(s)

The Change Calendar can be applied in any health care setting because of the universal impact of uncontrolled change on caregivers' ability to provide safe care. The specific application described in this article is within a Level 1 trauma center—Regions

Figure 1.
Current and Desired States of Change in a Health Care Organization

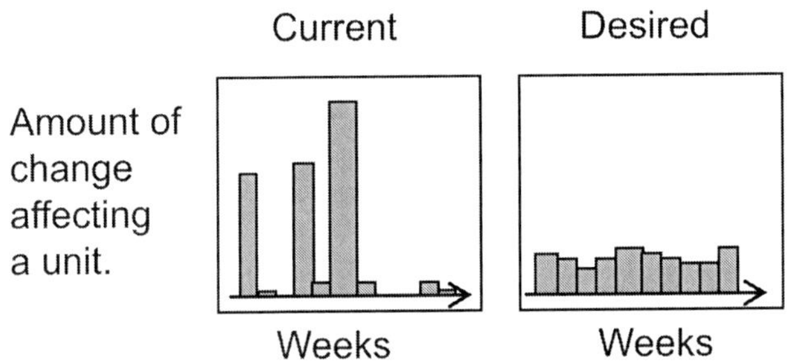

Source: Joint Commission Resources, 2007.

The Change Calendar is intended to help an organization make the transition from the periodic "avalanche" (left) to the future "snowfall" (right).

Hospital (St. Paul). The scope of the Change Calendar includes all changes faced by direct and indirect caregivers that potentially contribute to the cognitive factors already identified as endemic in health care and that thereby increase risks to patient safety (especially when they occur simultaneously).

The remainder of this article describes the use of the Change Calendar and provides lessons learned during its implementation at Regions Hospital, which began in December 2004 following its piloting at Childrens Hospitals and Clinics of Minnesota (Minneapolis/St. Paul).[6]

How To

The following "steps," as described for Regions Hospital, are not a sequential process but rather are independent tasks that can be done in parallel.

Step 1. Identify an Accountable Department

As an almost daily operational process, the Change Calendar must be managed by an accountable department, not a committee. The appropriate department will have the skills and the breadth and depth of organizational involvement required to manage the Change Calendar. In many organizations, the quality or performance improvement, Six Sigma department, or other group responsible for facilitating and supporting change, would be the logical choice. At Regions, the Change Calendar is maintained by the nursing educators and is routinely reviewed by the executive leadership and the board of trustees quality committee.

Step 2. Choose Software to Manage the Change Calendar

Commercially available project management software is available to meet the Change Calendar's requirements. Direct care units and ancillary departments are designated as the "resources." A unit's capacity for change, which is accumulated on a weekly basis, becomes constrained when it reaches 100%. Maintaining the calendar is time-consuming initially (that is, when creating an inventory of all initiatives) but reaches steady state (that is, the time when calendar updates become relatively constant) rather quickly.

Step 3. Control the Scope

Scope control applies to the Change Calendar, as it does for managing any program of projects. The three critical success factors for controlling calendar scope are as follows:

1. **Include all changes affecting direct/indirect caregivers.** Expectations about the Change Calendar must be managed from the beginning—emphasize that it applies only to changes affecting the sharp end of care. It was not to be used as the calendar of events for Regions, nor did it include management activities. In the pilot, local, unit-level changes were outside the scope of the Change Calendar. This decision was reversed during the pilot's first week because these local changes (for example, a unit competency effort) often either consumed the unit's total capacity for change, or a small change (for example, reading a short article on patient safety) put the unit into overload status when combined with a simultaneous organization-wide change (for example, reading and adapting to an urgent memo from The Joint Commission). Any change, no matter how "small", when combined with other changes, can result in "too much" change for a unit or department in a given week.
2. **Coordinate the timing.** It must be clear from the outset that the Change Calendar is intended to enhance patient safety by coordinating the timing of implementation of changes. It is not intended to serve the change management leadership functions of approving or prioritizing resources for improvement projects. Approval of the "quality agenda" (that is, which improvement initiatives are to be supported) is a separate organizational process that launches initiatives; it is the initiatives' implementation that is scheduled via the Change Calendar.
3. **The Change Calendar must start small and grow.** Implementing the Change Calendar is an evolutionary process. Design of all the project tasks does not need to be completed for implementation to begin. Regions successfully used

a four-task "middle-out" implementation approach, as follows:

- First, tap into existing structured change management processes (for example, information technology, facilities and materials management) and ensure that the implementation plans from these functions are captured in the calendar.
- Second, involve all managers, directors, and professional staff committees to create a common conceptual model and expectations.
- Third, expand to bottom-up awareness by capturing and documenting unit-level changes through the unit managers, nursing educators, and clinical nurse specialists.
- Fourth, once trust in the process and content is achieved at all organizational levels, use the Change Calendar proactively to schedule the timing of changes.

Step 4. Develop a Framework to Detect Changes and Estimate Degree of Impact

Detecting Changes. The initial challenge in creating the Change Calendar is determining the changes that must be included. The principal contributors to the calendar (that is, the dimensions of the calendar) are as follows:

- Information technology
- Competencies and education
- Policies and procedures
- Materials management
- Equipment
- Compliance
- Research
- Operational (for example, new residents every summer, new surgeons).

Assessing Degree of Impact. The next phase (which continues today at Regions on an ongoing basis) addresses how to estimate a change's impact on caregivers and patient safety. The challenge is to determine what mea-sure to use to create the unit-level aggregate impacts depicted in Figure 1. If Regions had taken a more traditional health care approach to this question, it could have taken years to research and develop an acceptable measurement tool. Rather than delay implementing the Change Calendar, Regions adapted a nursing education method to assess cognitive impact by using the "3 Cs" of curriculum design:

- Communication (awareness)
- Comprehension (understanding)
- Competency (skills)

Currently a simple rule of thumb is applied to these categories. For a specified week on each unit or in each indirect care department,

- Each communication change consumes 10% of an affected unit's capacity.
- Each comprehension change consumes 25% to 50% of an affected unit's capacity.
- Each competency change consumes 50% to 100% of an affected unit's capacity.

These percentages are added to yield the percentage of capacity forecast to be consumed on any given unit on any given week.

Output

A sample from Regions' Change Calendar is provided in Figure 2 (on page 139). Regions' long-range plan is to provide unit-level access to the read-only calendar via its intranet. When the evolution of the Change Calendar is complete, a unit will be able to view its forecasted changes by week for any specified date range. Until then, most of an organization's information needs are addressed in a semi-monthly tabular "snapshot" (Table 1, page 140) transcribed from the project management software file that forecasts "what's coming."

Results and Lessons Learned

Once the Change Calendar reaches sufficient accuracy and completeness to allow it to be used proactively to schedule changes, an additional benefit surfaces—it can be used to identify which units should be tapped for proof-of-concept and pilot efforts. This awareness of who is engaged in pilot efforts and who is available will help to prevent the burnout of units that have successfully performed pilot initiatives in the past.

Summary and Recommendations

The Change Calendar can be used to improve patient safety by smoothing the amount of change on any given unit on any given week. To be successful in implementing the Change Calendar, an organization must do the following:

1. Keep it simple.
2. Involve every level of the organization.
3. Manage the Change Calendar's scope by limiting it to changes that affect direct and indirect caregivers; do not include changes that apply to management (although a separate "blunt end" version could be adapted for managers and executives).
4. Identify a principal contact resource with sufficient breadth of awareness to manage the calendar.

Figure 2.
Sample Taken from the Change Calendar at Regions Hospital

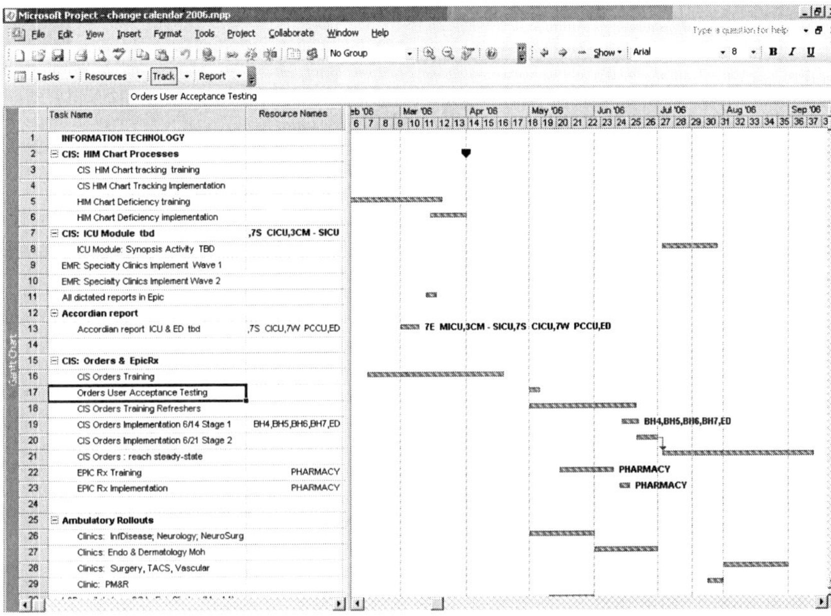

Source: Joint Commission Resources, 2007.

The sample depicts tasks for Orders User Acceptance Testing for the information technology unit at Regions Hospital, February–September 2006.

5. Manage staff expectations by educating them that the calendar is a tool to limit change fatigue and improve patient safety through timing and coordination of improvement initiatives.
6. Approach this task not as a project but rather as a culture change.
7. Organizations can simplify the measurement of the Change Calendar's impact by using two simple measures of success:
    - Is the calendar used to "clear" changes for several weeks around major implementations (for example, rollout of the electronic medical record)?
    - Does leadership ask: "Is this initiative on the Change Calendar?"

Table 1.
Monthly Change Calendar "Snapshot" for the Information Technology Unit*

Category	February	March	April
Information Technology	Epic CIS: • Orders: Superuser training • Chart Deficiency: CBT • Accordion report (ICUs & ED) training	Epic CIS: • Orders: training • Chart Deficiency: implement (12) • Accordion report (ICUs & ED) (1) (also available to all Regions users) • EpicRx training (pharmacy) Dictaphone: implement	Epic CIS: • Orders & EpicRx go-live (19) (ED, BH, L&D, nurses, pharmacists, HUCs) • Orders: Physician Training (for June 7 go live) • ICU Module: Synopsis Activity (19)
Education & Competencies	• Relationship Based Care (Wave 3: 8E, 8W, maternal-child cluster) • Handwashing (6S & Davita pilot) • Education Day (28)	• Compliant Documentation Management Program (CDMP; concurrent docu mentation review) (13) • Relationship Based Care (Wave 4) • Pressure ulcer surveillance (22) • Unit Practice Councils start	• CDMP • Relationship Based Care (Wave 4)
Policies & Procedures	• Joint Commission follow-up action items • Admission nurse in ED (pilot) • Pharmacist in ED for medication rec-onciliation (pilot)	• All dictation found on Epic (13th)	

Table 1. (continued)
Monthly Change Calendar "Snapshot" for the Information Technology Unit*

Equipment & Materials			
Facilities	• 5 South renovation • Mock Up New Facility Patient Room (17) • NICU relocates Feb 20th	• 5 South renovation	• 5 South Renovation to July 20
Compliance	• JCAHO follow-up report		
Research			
Operational	• HR Employee Survey (13)		

*As transcribed from the project management software file that forecasts "what's coming"

CIS: clinical information system; CBT, computer-based training; ICU, intensive care unit; ED, emergency department; BH, behavioral health; L&D, labor and delivery; HUCs, health unit coordinators; CDMP, concurrent data management program (concurrent documentation to support accurate coding); NICU, neonatal ICU; HR, human resources

Source: Joint Commission Resources, 2007.

This article originally appeared in The Joint Commission Journal on Quality and Patient Safety, June 2007, vol. 33, No. 6.

References

1. Kotter J.P.: *Leading Change.* Boston: Harvard Business School Press, 1996.

2. Beaudan E.: Making change last: How to get beyond change fatigue. *Ivey Business Journal*, Jan.–Feb 2006. http://www.iveybusiness journal.com/view_article.asp?intArticle_ID=608 (last accessed Apr. 17, 2007).

3. Scott-Morgan P., et al: *The End of Change: How Your Company Can Sustain Growth and Innovation While Avoiding Change Fatigue.* New York: McGraw Hill, 2001.

4. Simpson K.R., Knox E.G.: Adverse perinatal outcomes. Recognizing, understanding and preventing common accidents. *AWHONN Lifelines* 7:224–235, Jun.–Jul. 2003.

5. Valusek J.R.: Personal interviews with nursing educators at Regions Hospital, St. Paul, Jan. 2005.

6. Valusek J.R., Morath J.M.: Change: Dealing with a root cause of patient safety accidents. Paper presented at the First Safety Across High-Consequence Industries Conference, Parks College of Engineering and Aviation and School of Public Health, at St. Louis University, St. Louis, Mar. 9, 2004.

Index

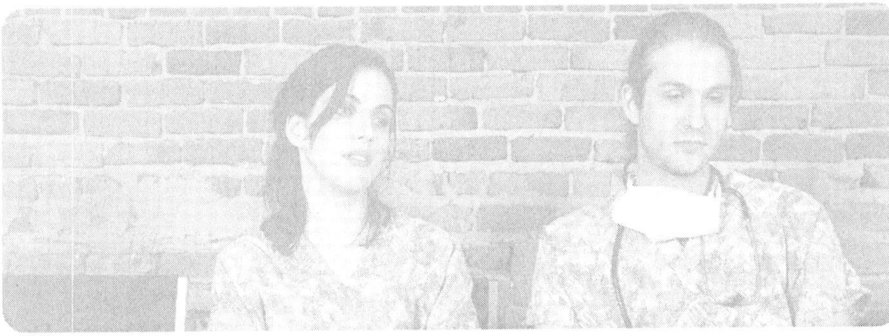

T